/M/ AMERICAN *MARKETING* ASSOCIATION

Marketing
ENCYCLOPEDIA

Issues and Trends
Shaping the Future

Jeffrey Heilbrunn
Editor

Printed on recyclable paper

American Marketing Association
Chicago, Illinois

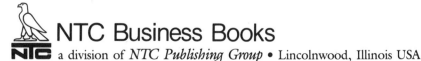

NTC Business Books
a division of *NTC Publishing Group* • Lincolnwood, Illinois USA

Library of Congress Cataloging-in-Publication Data

AMA marketing encyclopedia : issues and trends shaping the future /
   American Marketing Association : Jeffrey Heilbrunn, editor.
      p.   cm.
   Includes index.
   ISBN 0-8442-3593-8
   1. Marketing—Encyclopedias.   I. Heilbrunn, Jeffrey.
II. American Marketing Association.
HF5415.A46   1995
658′.003—dc20
                                                     94-17747
                                                        CIP

Published in conjunction with the American Marketing Association,
250 South Wacker Drive, Chicago, Illinois 60606.

1996 Printing

Published by NTC Business Books, a division of NTC Publishing Group
© 1995 by NTC Publishing Group, 4255 West Touhy Avenue,
Lincolnwood (Chicago), Illinois 60646-1975 U.S.A.
Manufactured in the United States of America

5 6 7 8 9 BC 9 8 7 6 5 4 3 2

Contents

Section V
Strategic Marketing Management   163

Section VI
Micromarkets and Micromarketing   239

Section VII
Information Collection and Analysis   275

Foreword

Marketing: From Transactions to Mutual Loyalty

The American Marketing Association defines marketing as "the process of using the marketing mix (price, product, promotion and place) to bring about transactions of items of value between two or more parties." This definition focuses on the traditional activities of a marketing department, whose goal is to bring about discrete tranactions. But marketing is more than just the next sale.

The strategic form of marketing redefines marketing's goal in terms of customer astisfaction. The company strategy is to continuously acquire, satisfy, and retain customers for repeated transactions. In the department, marketing manipulates the famous 4 Ps of traditional marketing: price, product, promotion, and place (distribution). In strategic marketing, the four Ps of marketing are product, people, process, and progress.

Effective management of these elements, with the goal being customer satisfaction—the meeting and exceeding of customer expectations—will lead to loyal customers. Loyal customers are ones with whom we can build an ongoing personal relationship. This in turn breeds employee satisfaction . . . a self-feeding, positive system of growth. The opposite, customer and employee dissatisfaction, can create the opposite effect, a doom loop.

Driving customer satisfaction can be accomplished in many ways, but it all must start with the basic tenet of marketing:

KNOW THY CUSTOMER

From here, the possibilities to satisfy and delight are perhaps endless. New technologies, and new insights, and new personnel policies are all in play.

There are so many roads to customer satisfaction and effective marketing that no one can possibly travel all of them, even though we are all constantly in search of the silver bullet that will impress our customers and give us a leg up on the competition.

Keeping Up

This book has been developed to help you catch up with the hottest concepts that you can use to find, satisfy, and keep customers. Each contribution to this unique and authoritative work is written by a leading authority associated with the contribution. Use this book as an update course in marketing; use it as a source of ideas; use it as a way to constantly challenge your thinking about how you do business. And if you need a more in-depth treatment of a topic, you are encouraged to seek out the works of our notable contributors.

Acknowledgments

This volume includes contributions from 50 leading experts in both traditional and leading-edge marketing concepts. I thank them all for their special contributions to this work. I also wish to thank the Office of the Chairperson of the Board of Directors of AMA for their support and encouragement in bringing about this project.

Most of all, I thank you for buying this book. I hope it will be the beginning of a long relationship, not a one-time transaction.

Jeffrey Heilbrunn
Crystal Lake, Illinois

Section I

New Products and Services

New products have traditionally been the lifeblood of successful enterprises as well as the most risky area of marketing. With the increased costs of development the potential risks—and rewards—have increased exponentially. In this section leading authorities discuss how product managers of the future will meet the challenges of developing new products.

In "New Product Development: New Approaches for the New Marketplace," Thomas D. Kuczmarski discusses a new "disciplined freedom" to create products that meet the needs of an ever-changing, fractionalized marketplace. In "Mass Customization: Emerging Techniques for Emerging Markets," B. Joseph Pine II surveys the new techniques being developed to tailor products that meet the needs and demands of individual customers. The rise of environmental concerns and their impact on organizations is the subject of the next two articles, "Strategies for Making Green a Competitive Edge," by Jacquelyn Ottman and "Enviropreneurial Marketing," by P. Rajan Varadarajan. Ottman identifies practical strategies that marketers can use to respond to the growing numbers of consumers who are swayed by the impact that products have on the environment. From a different perspective Varadarajan discusses how organizations can create progressive management policies and procedures that will nurture "green" corporate cultures and foster creative approaches to products and markets. And in "Meeting the Supervalue Challenge," Philip Kotler focuses on the consumer who expects "more for less" and how the supervalue marketers of the present will be the big winners of the future.

1

–1–
NEW PRODUCT DEVELOPMENT
New Approaches for the New Marketplace

Thomas D. Kuczmarski

Thomas D. Kuczmarski is president and founder of the Chicago-based consulting firm Kuczmarski & Associates, recently named one of North America's "100 Leading Management Consulting Firms" by *Consultants News*. He is an expert on innovation, growth management strategies, and new product development. He is regularly quoted and published in leading magazines and newspapers such as *The Wall Street Journal, Fortune, Newsweek,* and *USA Today.*

New product development is the process of commercializing a new idea or concept into a marketable product or service. New products and services can be developed in a systematic way if managers apply a disciplined process that is understood and consistently used by all functional areas within a company.

The Development Process: A Ten-Step Approach

Companies use a variety of approaches to develop new products. Although no single process is suited for all companies, there are common elements of effective processes that serve as guideposts for constructing a company-specific new product process. The traditional process should be adapted to your own company culture and objectives. The ten-step development process shown in Figure 1 offers a logical, systematic, and well-tested approach for taking a set of potential market or need categories and generating ideas from them which will eventually evolve into commercialized new products.

The ten steps of the new product development process are:

1. *Needs-and-wants exploration.* Examine external market and competitive trends, ascertain potential needs and wants of each customer segment, and identify problems that customers cite.

2. *Idea generation.* Through a variety of problem-solving and creative approaches, generate new ideas that fit the identified categories.

3 *Concept development.* Take ideas that pass initial screens and develop a three-dimensional description of the product.

4. *Business analysis.* For each concept, formulate a market and competitive assessment that leads to a pro forma for two to three years.

5. *Screening.* Keeping in mind financial forecasts developed in the business analysis, pass the remaining concepts through all performance criteria.

Futurescope

The new products of the 21st century will be developed using a problem-solving approach that takes into account the diversity of customer wants and needs. The information about consumers' wants, needs, complaints, and problems will be gathered in increasingly specific detail from electronic and traditional sources. New product managers will need to be knowledgeable about specialized market niches in order to bring exciting new services and products into an ever-changing, fractionalized marketplace.

Figure 1 Ten-Step Development Process

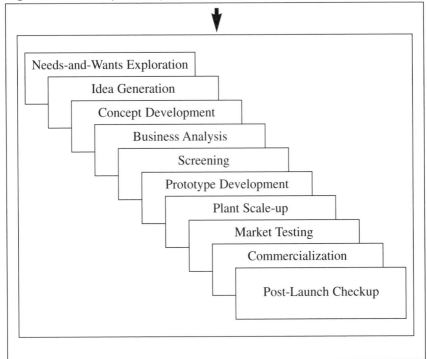

Needs-and-Wants Exploration
Idea Generation
Concept Development
Business Analysis
Screening
Prototype Development
Plant Scale-up
Market Testing
Commercialization
Post-Launch Checkup

6. *Prototype development.* Complete development of product and run product-performance tests.

7. *Plant scale-up and manufacturing testing.* Determine rollout equipment needs and manufacture product in large enough quantities to identify bugs and problems. Run product-performance tests.

8. *Market testing.* Determine consumer purchase intent. Test the product in either a simulated market or actual market rollout.

9. *Commercialization.* Introduce the product to the trade and consumers.

10. *Post-launch checkup.* Monitor performance of the new product six and twelve months after launch relative to original forecasts. After one year, performance is monitored annually.

One important aspect of developing new products successfully is to understand that problem solving should drive idea generation. This means that the first step, needs-and-wants exploration, provides the foundation and platform for effective idea generation. This step should surface needs, wants, gripes, complaints, and problems that customers have about a certain activity, function, or product performance. Innovative new products should be developed to solve either perceived or real needs, wants, or problems of customers.

Thus, successful companies have a systematic and orderly process with sequential steps in place that guide the development of an idea into a commercialized new product. Using the same process uniformly yields the most product results. A new product development process provides a thinking and action framework for transforming new product objectives into new products that are successful in the market.

Organizing for New Product Development

New product development is a complex and subtle process. It can be accomplished using a step-by-step approach, because it blends creativity with analytics. However, it is still more of an art than a science. Consequently, having a systematic process alone is not enough. Success depends on how well a company implements the process.

Companies need to make a long-term commitment to new products by providing the necessary funds and managerial know-how. Importantly, top management needs to make a visible commitment to this endeavor by establishing the right organization structure, staffed with the most qualified people tied together with an effective incentive and reward system.

The best organization for new products is most often a stand-alone "department" that reports directly to senior management and is staffed with dedicated managers. However, when full-time new product people cannot be allocated for a free-standing new product structure, a multidisciplinary team that draws on different functional managers can be effective. The team approach encourages interaction of various skilled resources, facilitates decision making, and stimulates commitment across functional departments throughout the development process.

A single manager should coordinate the new products process. This person should have total accountability and be responsible for marshaling new product activities. The skills required of a new product manager rest more on effectiveness in motivating people, listening, and following through with details than on any specific functional or technical expertise. Beyond effective people-handling skills, a new products manager must have strong analytical acumen, be a risk-taker and a product champion, and have entrepreneurial instincts and a sense of vision. Being a persuasive and motivating communicator caps the essential ingredients of a new products manager.

Finally, giving new product participants some latitude and creative freedom often generates a greater degree of innovation. But there must be a balance between structure and flexibility and between teamwork and individual accomplishment. A term I've coined, *disciplined freedom,* describes a management style that provides balance between giving individuals a sense of entrepreneurship and creativity and providing enough control and direction to guide their efforts.

—2—

MASS CUSTOMIZATION

An Emerging Model for Emerging Markets

B. Joseph Pine II

B. Joseph Pine II is the founder and president of Ridgefield, Connecticut-based Strategic Horizons, Inc., a management consulting firm specializing in helping companies envision and then realize their futures. Mr. Pine is the author of the highly acclaimed book *Mass Customization: The New Frontier in Business Competition,* which *The Financial Times* named one of the top business books of 1993. In it he details the historic shift from mass production to mass customization—the low-cost, high-quality creation of individually customized goods and services. He has also written articles for a number of magazines and journals, including the *Harvard Business Review, The Wall Street Journal, Planning Review,* the *IBM Systems Journal, Chief Executive,* and *CIO.*

As a business model, mass production was tremendously successful throughout most of the 20th century. As depicted in Figure 1, mass production revolved around a company taking a new product and finding the one best way to produce it, yielding standardized products at a low cost and generally of consistent quality. These were sold into large, homogeneous markets (and often helped create those markets), which provided the company with stable demand levels and afforded it long product life cycles and long development cycles. Every once in a while, a new product would emerge that would be worth the high changeover costs, and the cycle would repeat. (Although manufacturing terms are used, the same basic process holds true for many service industries, particularly insurance and other financial services.)

Mass production is the search for efficiency through stability and control. As long as markets are stable and inputs, processes, and outputs can be controlled, then it can work effectively. However, when companies find that what they began developing years ago and produced weeks or months ago can no longer be reliably sold today—when markets are uncertain, unstable and unpredictable—then mass production simply no longer works. No amount of microtargeting or micropositioning will provide any lasting advantage when the rest of the organization acts anything like the model shown in Figure 1.

Rather, companies have to take this feedback loop and reverse it, as depicted in Figure 2. Instead of reinforcing on longer cycle times, greater standardization, and more homogeneity—which no longer exists—the opposite occurs. Increasingly heterogeneous markets demand not only low cost and high quality but also increasing customization. This requires the firm to develop new mass-customization processes, out of which flow new products that must be rapidly developed,

Futurescope

Mass customization is the low-cost, high-quality delivery of individually customized goods and services. It is a new business model that makes identifying and fulfilling individual customer wants and needs paramount within the organization. Mass customization is emerging today but will be in full force in many industries by the year 2000. Mass customization is not microsegmentation, niche marketing, micromarketing, database marketing, or any other technique that targets messages and positionings to individuals. These techniques can be usefully employed by mass customizers, but usually these techniques are the dying gasps of mass producers finding it impossible to compete in increasingly turbulent markets.

Figure 1   Mass Production As a Dynamic System

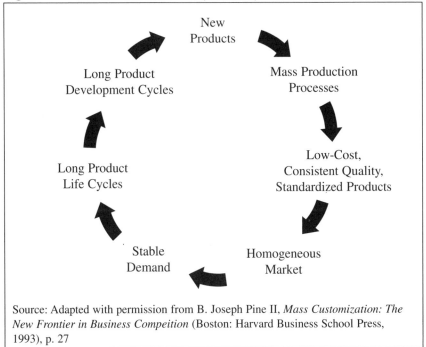

Source: Adapted with permission from B. Joseph Pine II, *Mass Customization: The New Frontier in Business Compeition* (Boston: Harvard Business School Press, 1993), p. 27

for they will have short product life cycles, which helps to further fragment demand, leading to even greater heterogeneity, and so on.

The end result? An entire organization geared around the fulfillment of individual customer wants and needs. An organization where not only messages are targeted to individuals, but also products are tailored and made to order. An organization where everyone is responsible for marketing in its truest sense: creating customers and fulfilling their desires. But also an organization that realizes the competitive and customer imperatives for low cost and high quality.

Although no one has embraced mass customization in the same sense that first Ford and then General Motors can be said to have perfected mass production, many companies are coming close. Perhaps the closest is Motorola, and its Paging Products Group in particular. The company's sales reps go into a customer's office with a laptop computer, and together they design the set of pagers that exactly meet that customer's needs (out of 29 million possibilities). The pager designs are then immediately transmitted through to the factory floor, where an almost fully automated, lot-size-of-one flexible manufacturing system can produce them in a matter of hours for shipment that day or the next.

One of the premier service companies to embrace mass customization is the United Services Automobile Association. Based on events that happen in each

Figure 2 A New Paradigm of Mass Customization

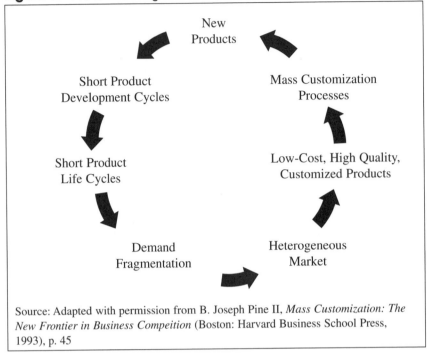

Source: Adapted with permission from B. Joseph Pine II, *Mass Customization: The New Frontier in Business Compeition* (Boston: Harvard Business School Press, 1993), p. 45

member's life, USAA customizes its growing portfolio of services. Typically for a mass customizer, it has expanded beyond insurance to other financial services and even to consumer goods. Whether customers are getting married, having a baby, or buying a car, USAA is determined to have the exact set of products and services each of its members needs during those major life events.

Mass customization is not an oxymoron. As Motorola, USAA, and many other companies have discovered, it is a completely new way of doing business that may be the only means of achieving sustained success in increasingly turbulent markets.

—3—

STRATEGIES FOR MAKING GREEN A COMPETITIVE EDGE

Jacquelyn A. Ottman

Jacquelyn A. Ottman is the president of J. Ottman Consulting, Inc., a strategic resource management company that she founded in 1989 to advise forward-thinking companies on the development and promotion of environmentally sound products. Her clients include Colgate-Palmolive, Kraft General Foods, DuPont, General Electric, and Eastman-Kodak. A pioneer in environmental marketing, Ms. Ottman is the creator of the *Getting to Zero*[sm] process, the first concept-generation process specifically designed for environment-related new product invention. She is author of the award-winning book, *Green Marketing: Challenges and Opportunities for the New Marketing Age,* and a co-author of *Environmental Consumerism: What Every Marketer Needs to Know* and *Green Marketing Anthology.* She also is a featured columnist for *American Marketplace* and *Marketing News,* and is a sought-after speaker at conferences in the United States and abroad.

11

Just a few years ago, superconcentrated laundry detergents gathered dust in a Denver test market. Paper towels made from recycled content were rejected as inferior, even unclean. And bulky packaging added perceived value to consumer products. More was more, whiter was better, and disposability was king. But all of this is rapidly changing. A new marketing age has arrived.

Challenges and Opportunities of Greening

From now on, companies that don't respond to "green" issues with safer and more environmentally sound products risk falling out of sync with the consumer. And for marketers who do heed the consumer's call, opportunities abound. Sales at Church & Dwight, makers of Arm & Hammer baking soda, have grown from $16 million to $500 million thanks in part to a timely and thorough response to the trend. Concentrated laundry products cut down on waste and are more profitable than full-strength alternatives. With a product that is kinder to the environment as well as to people, 3M has expanded the market for paint strippers.

While the opportunities are enormous, so too are the challenges. Among them:

- No clear-cut methodology exists for comparing the environmental impacts of one product against another.

- Most consumers are reluctant to make trade-offs in their life-styles and product purchasing in their quest for a cleaner planet.

- Misperceptions abound, representing the potential for unproductive public policymaking and significant risks to industry in the form of unnecessary and costly changes in products and manufacturing processes.

Futurescope

With garbage piling up in our communities, old-growth forests disappearing at an alarming rate, and the air getting harder to breathe, a revolution is underway to halt the misuse of our planet's resources. This revolution is taking place at our nation's supermarkets, drug stores, and mass merchandisers. To the growing legions of consumers concerned about the quality of their lives and the lives of their children, "less" is now becoming "more," and purchasing decisions are increasingly being swayed by the impact that products have on the environment.

- There are no national uniform guidelines for communicating commonly used environmental marketing terms. The FTC has issued voluntary guidelines for terms such as *recycled, recyclable,* and *biodegradable,* but these are not legally enforceable, and they do not preempt stricter guidelines put forth by states such as New York, California, and Rhode Island. Without uniform guidelines, the environmental messages of national marketers cannot be heard, and the potential to confuse consumers is great.

- Industry is seen as the key contributor to environmental blight, and, as a result, it has low credibility in communicating environment-related messages. A backlash from skeptical environmentalists, regulators, and the press is already in place.

Strategies for Success

The companies that stand to gain the most from consumers' environmentalism will adopt a *proactive response* to the issues, integrating environmental planning into overall business strategy. They will develop products that balance consumer's concerns for performance/quality, convenience, and affordability with minimal environmental impact. And they will communicate their environmental initiatives to all corporate stakeholders with credibility, enlisting third-party support as necessary.

As a critical first step in overall corporate greening, successful marketers will green their companies before greening their marketing activities. As Hubert H. "Skip" Humphrey III, Attorney General of Minnesota and principal author of the landmark document, *Green Report II* has said, "Green your operations and the products will take care of themselves. Green your products and the marketing will take care of itself."

Following are ten strategies that forward-thinking, committed companies can use to ensure continued markets for their products, and an abundance of opportunities to leverage environmental strategies as a source of competitive advantage.

Ten Winning Strategies for Succeeding in the Age of Environmental Consumerism[1]

1. Do Your Homework

- Understand the full range of environmental, economic, political, and social issues that affect your business.

[1]Reprinted with permission from *Green Marketing: Challenges and Opportunities for the New Marketing Age* (Lincolnwood, Ill.: NTC Business Books, 1993).

2. Get Your House in Order

- Green from the top down as well as the bottom up:
  - Start with a commitment from the CEO.
  - Empower employees to develop environmentally sound products and processes
- Enlist the support of independent auditors.
- Integrate environmental issues into marketing planning.
- Turn your brand managers into "brand stewards," responsible for achieving corporate profit objectives with minimal environmental and social impact. Require an environmental assessment in all business reviews.
- Communicate your corporate commitment and project your values.

3. Be a Leader

- Be proactive; set standards for your industry.
- Foster cooperation among your competitors.

4. Build Coalitions with Corporate Environmental Stakeholders

- Educate consumers on environmental issues and how to solve them. Help teachers educate our young.
- Work with legislators and governmental agencies to develop balanced legislation and regulations.
- Share information with environmental groups and solicit their technical support.
- Inform the media of your environmental initiatives.
- Help retailers address consumer needs and reduce waste through the creation of special promotional programs and cosponsored recycling programs.

5. Develop Products that Balance Consumers' Needs

- Combine high quality, convenience, and affordable pricing with environmental soundness.
- Minimize the environmental impact of products and packaging at every stage of the product life cycle.
- Take the high road. Strive to use leading-edge technologies, materials, and design. Source reduce, i.e., use fewer materials or toxics, whenever possible.

6. Empower Consumers

- Help consumers understand the environmental benefits of your products and packaging.

- Address the diversity of green. Reward environmentally active consumers for their commitment and motivate passive green consumers with easy, cost-effective substitutes for existing products.

7. Underpromise and Overdeliver on Your Environmental Marketing Claims.

- In keeping with the voluntary guidelines recommended by the Federal Trade Commission, don't overstate, exaggerate, or mislead consumers.

- Use claims that are specific and supported by reliable, scientific evidence.

8. Establish Credibility

- Position product initiatives as part of your ongoing commitment to the environment.

- Use third parties such as environmental groups, regulators, and educators to add credibility and impact to your messages.

- Promote responsible consumption of your products.

9. Minimize the Environmental Impact of Your Marketing Programs

- Use recycled paper and vegetable-based inks. Cut down on unnecessary mailings. Print on both sides of paper.

10. Think Long Term

- Adapt to shifts in consumer attitudes, legislative trends, and changes in natural resources availability.

For Further Reading

American Marketplace. Bi-monthly newsletter. Business Publishers, Inc., Silver Spring, MD.

Business Ethics Magazine. Marjorie Kelly, ed. Mavis Publications, Minneapolis, MN.

Conservation Directory of Environmental Organizations. National Wildlife Federation, Washington, DC.

Design for Recycling: A Plastic Bottle Recycler's Perspective. Richard A. Fleming. Partnership for Plastics Progress, The Society of the Plastics Industry, Washington, DC.

Design for the Environment. Dorothy Mackenzie. Rizzoli International Publications, New York, NY.

DMA Environmental Resource for Direct Marketers. Direct Marketing Association, New York, NY, 1990.

Environmental Almanac. World Resources Institute, Houghton Mifflin, Boston, MA, 1992.

Green Company Resource Guide: Leading Resources for Environmentally Sound Business. The New Consumer Institute, Wauconda, IL.

Green MarketAlert. Monthly newsletter. MarketAlert Publications, Bethlehem, CT.

Green 2000. Monthly packaging newsletter. Packaging Strategies, West Chester, PA.

In Business. Magazine for environmental entrepreneurs. Jerome Goldstein, ed. The JG Press, Inc., Emmaus, PA.

Shopping for a Better World: A Quick and Easy Guide to Socially Responsible Supermarket Shopping. Ben Corson, et al. Council on Economic Priorities, New York, NY, 1992.

State of the World. Lester Brown, et al. World Watch, W.W. Norton, New York, NY, 1992.

State Recycling Laws Update. Raymond Communications, Riverdale, MD, 1992.

—4—

ENVIROPRENEURIAL MARKETING

P. Rajan Varadarajan

Rajan Varadarajan is Foley's Professor of Retailing and Marketing at Texas A&M University and editor of the *Journal of Marketing*. Dr. Varadarajan's interests are corporate, business, and marketing strategy; marketing management; and global competitive strategy. He is author of more than 60 refereed journal articles and is co-author of *Contemporary Perspectives on Strategic Market Planning*. Dr. Varadarajan received his M.A. in industrial management from the Indian Institute of Technology, Madras, India, and his Ph.D. in business administration from the University of Massachusetts, Amherst.

The concept of *green marketing* entered the business lexicon in the late 1980s, soon to be followed by equivalent terms such as *environmental marketing* and *enviropreneurial marketing* and related concepts such as the *environmental entrepreneur, ecopreneur,* and *enviropreneur.* Although there are some differences in the way these concepts are defined by different authors, for the most part they are generally built around the following themes:

- **Enviropreneur:** A person who in organizing and assuming the risks and managing the activities of a business enterprise (i.e., an entrepreneur) explores market opportunities for environment-friendly products, processes, and technologies and pursues environmentally responsible policies, procedures, and practices. (Other terms used interchangeably: *environmental entrepreneur* and *ecopreneur.*)

- **Enviropreneurial firms:** Organizations that pursue environmentally responsible policies, procedures, and practices in the conduct of their business activities. (Other term used interchangeably: environmentally oriented firms.)

- **Enviropreneurial managers:** Executives who champion the adoption of environmentally responsible policies, procedures, and practices by the various organizational units of the firm they are affiliated with.

- **Enviropreneurial marketing:** Environmentally responsible policies, strategies, and tactics initiated by a firm in the realm of marketing in order to achieve a competitive differentiation advantage for the firm's offerings vis-à-vis competitor's offerings, and/or influenced by the firm's progressive views on the duties and responsibilities of a corporate citizen. (Other terms used interchangeably: green marketing and environmental marketing.)

Futurescope

With the dawn of green consumerism—a growing preference among consumers for goods and services that are environment friendly—there seems to be little doubt that pursuit of ecologically responsible and environmentally friendly policies and practices across the entire spectrum of an organization's activities is likely to become an increasingly important organizational imperative in the years ahead. Inasmuch as innovation, entrepreneurship, and intrapreneurship are critical to the survival, growth, and profitability of organizations, nurturing a corporate culture conducive to the pursuit of progressive enviropreneurial management policies and practices is likely to become critical in upholding an organization's legitimacy in the eyes of stakeholders.

It is evident from an examination of the extensive coverage of this phenomenon in the business press as well as the popular press that enviropreneurship and enviropreneurial marketing are taking deep roots in a growing number of organizations, as well as gradually gaining consumer acceptance.

As detailed in Table 1, the driving forces underlying this movement—including sociocultural, legal-regulatory-political, competitive, and, most importantly, international organizational forces—seem to be gaining in momentum. Furthermore, in recent years, numerous companies have been signatories to the Valdez Principles, contestants in the annual competition for the Edison Awards for Environmental Achievement, and participants in the evaluation processes designed to independently test products for environmental certification programs such as the Green Cross and Green Seal. Table 2 provides an overview of these recent phenomena.

Characteristics of Green Products

There seems to be a general recognition that the greenness of a product is a matter of degree, relative to the competing alternatives available, and that considerable variance can exist regarding acceptable levels of greenness across product categories, as well as within a product category across countries (see Ottman). Nevertheless, there also appears to be some consensus in regard to the dimensions along which improvements in a product contribute to its relative greenness. For instance, Elkington, Hailes, and Makower list the following as the ideal characteristics of green products:

- Are not dangerous to people or animals
- Do not damage the environment in manufacture, use, or disposal
- Do not consume a disproportionate amount of energy in manufacture, use, or disposal
- Do not cause unnecessary waste
- Do not involve unnecessary cruelty to animals
- Do not use materials from threatened species or environments.

Corporate Responses to the Environmental Challenge

As detailed below, corporate responses to the environmental challenge have ranged from doing nothing to a proactive integrated corporate response.

1. Do nothing. Ignore the concerns of various stakeholders. Hope that the forces underlying the environmental movement are transient and will fade away.

Table 1 Environmental Forces Underlying Enviropreneurial Initiatives

Attractiveness of Market Environment

Size and rate of growth of market for end-use products that are environment friendly, as well as intermediate products, processes, and technologies employed in the manufacture of environment-friendly products.

Long-term adverse profit implications of not being proactive in developing environment-friendly products, processes, and technologies

Competitive Environment

Potential for achieving a sustainable competitive advantage

Basis for achieving a differentiation advantage in an era of me-too products

Need to neutralize the differentiation advantage achieved by a competitor pursuing environment-friendly policies and practices

Legal, Regulatory, and Political Environment

Recognition of impending threats (legal, regulatory, and political) due to growing concerns regarding the impact of the firm's product offerings on the environment

Reactive responses to (a) enacted or impending legislation and (b) directives or threat of action by regulatory bodies

Proactive responses designed to ward off new legislative and/or regulatory developments

Socio-cultural Environment

Growing environmental awareness and concern among the general public

Extensive coverage by media of impending and actual environmental disasters

Increase in the membership, wealth, and sophistication of pro-environment pressure groups

Internal Organizational Environment

Employee attitudes and expectations in the realm of progressive corporate practices relating to the environment, shaped by genuine concern for the wellness of the environment.

Potential for transfer of organizational learning from product categories and country markets where firms face more stringent governmental regulations and/or consumer expectations than other product categories and geographic markets

Sources: P. Rajan Varadarajan, "Marketing's Contribution to the Strategy Dialogue: The View from a Different Looking Glass," *Journal of the Academy of Marketing Science* 20 (Fall 1992), 335–344. Ken Peattie and Moire Ratnayaka, "Responding to the Green Movement," *Industrial Marketing Management*, 21 (1992), 103–110.

Table 2   Environmental Achievement Awards and Environmental
Seals of Approval: An Overview

The Valdez Principles

A set of principles designed by the Coalition for Environmentally Responsible Economies (CRES), a nonprofit membership organization, to promote environmentally responsible economic activity throughout the world. Companies that are signatories of the Valdez Principles agree to follow procedures and policies that adhere to the protection of the environment, including the following:

- Sustainable use of natural resources

- Reduction and disposal of wastes

- Wise use of energy

- Annual environmental audits

Awards for Environmental Achievement

The Edison Awards for Environmental Achievement are given to consumer products introduced since October 1992 that demonstrate significant achievements in the realms of source reduction and/or recycling. The winners of the annual award are chosen by an independent "green chip" panel of judges.

Environmental Seals of Approval: Certification and Labelling Programs

Two nonprofit organizations, the Green Cross Certification Co., Oakland, California, and Green Seal, Washington D.C., have come out with certification programs. Both programs set standards, test products, and award seals of approval. They are in their formative stages and are currently limited to a few product categories. For instance, among other requirements, in order to qualify for the Green Cross environmental seal, a product and its packaging must contain at least 50 percent recycled or sustainable materials, and manufacturers must eliminate all plant emissions that are carcinogenic or cause reproductive damage. The Green Seal label of approval certifies products found to be environmentally preferable on the basis of the environmental impact of the full life cycle of the product from raw materials and manufacturing through consumer use and recycling or disposal.

Sources: Eric R. Anderson, "Going Green: The Corporate Push for Environmental Consciousness," *Business Credit* (January 1992), 14–17. Michael Sansolo, "Going Green: Three Ways to Build Trust," *Progressive Grocer* (February 1992), 99, 45–50.

2. Defend present products, policies, and practices. Dispute damaging evidence, lobby to ward off impending legislation, and stress higher cost to customers of changing products, policies, and practices.

3. Symbolic response. Sponsor green events, contribute to the green movement, and express concerns over threat to the environment, but make no changes in products, policies, or practices.

4. Selective response. Respond only when customer demands and the lobbying by pressure groups are intense or the cost of noncompliance is prohibitive.

5. Reactive response. Modify product, packaging, and promotion in response to actions of competitors.

6. Proactive integrated corporate response. A corporate commitment to environmental orientation grounded in analysis and understanding of the marketing, manufacturing, and R&D initiatives that would enable a firm to effectively and proactively respond to the environmental challenge.

   A. **The marketing challenge:** What do customers want us to make? How will they use, reuse, or dispose of our offerings and when?

   B. **The manufacturing challenge:** How do we make, store, deliver, maintain, recycle, and dispose of our products, components, and materials?

   C. **The R&D challenge:** What products, processes, and materials technologies are needed to respond to the environmental challenge?

Promoting Environmental Sensitivity in Organizations

Although currently there seems to be considerable breadth and diversity in corporate responses to the environmental movement, the various forces underlying the environmental movement summarized in Table 1 suggest that in the near future the pursuit of environmentally responsible policies and practices is likely to increasingly become a corporate imperative, rather than an area where firms have considerable leeway. Elkington lists a number of activities conducive to promoting environmental sensitivity across the entire organization:

1. Developing and publishing an environmental strategy

2 Preparing an action program

3. Leading from the top, reflecting green concerns throughout the firm

4. Allocating adequate resources

5. Investing in environmental science and technology

6. Educating and training

7. Monitoring, auditing, and reporting

8. Monitoring the evolution of the green agenda

9. Contributing to environmental programs

10. Helping build bridges between the various interest groups

Perils of Exploiting
the Environmental Movement

In an era of me-too products, an increasing number of firms have come to recognize that environment-friendly product attributes can be a basis for differentiating their offerings from competitors' offerings. However, there have been instances of firms engaging in questionable practices in the realm of eniviropreneurial marketing. A task force report on responsible environmental advertising, *The Green Report,* cautions about two potential outcomes if current environmental marketing abuses continue.

1. If consumers begin to feel that their genuine interest in the environment is being exploited and rebel in response, they would no longer seek out or demand products that are in fact less damaging to the environment. If this were to occur, the environmental improvements that would have been achieved would be lost.

2. The tone, content, and number of environmental claims might lead the public to believe that specific environmental problems have been adequately addressed. This, in turn, could actually impede finding real solutions to identified problems by causing consumers to set aside their environmental concerns, making the assumption that these concerns had been addressed (see Davis, p. 14).

To date, a number of guidelines have been advanced in order to help firms to critically evaluate their eniviropreneurial marketing activities and the truthfulness of their advertising claims. For instance, Davis provides a detailed discussion on the following guidelines for the development of green marketing claims:

1, Conservatively interpret existing FTC and other legal guidelines.

2. Be specific about where the environmental benefit in the product or service lies.

3. Be specific about environmental benefits and provide definitional support.

Among the recommendations presented in *The Green Report II: Recommendations for Responsible Environmental Advertising,* a report of a task force of attorneys general representing eleven states, are the following:

- Environmental claims should be a specific as possible, and not general, vague, incomplete, or overly broad.

- Environmental claims relating to disposability should clearly disclose the general availability of the advertising option where the product is sold.

- Environmental claims should be substantive.

- Environmental claims should be supported by competent and reliable scientific evidence.

As organizations move into an era that is often characterized as the "green decade," close cooperation and interaction among the marketing, manufacturing, R&D, and purchasing personnel of an organization are critical to the successful development and introduction of products that possess environmentally sensitive product and packaging characteristics, are manufactured in an environmentally responsible manner, and are marketed in accordance with generally accepted guidelines.

References

Anderson, Eric R., "Going Green: The corporate Push for Environmental Consciousness," *Business Credit* (January 1992), 14–17.

Coddington, Walter. *Environmental Marketing: Positive Strategies for Reaching the Green Consumer.* New York: McGraw-Hill, 1993.

Davis, Joel J., "A Blueprint for Green Marketing," *The Journal of Business Strategy* 12 (July-August 1991), 14–17.

Elkington, John. *The Green Capitalists.* London: Victor Gollanz, 1989.

Elkington, John, Julie Hailes, and Joel Makower. *The Green Consumer.* New York: Penguin, 1990.

Ottman, Jacquelyn A. *Green Marketing.* Lincolnwood, Ill.: NTC Business Books, 1993.

Peattie, Ken, and Moire Ratnayaka, "Responding to the Green Movement," *Industrial Marketing Management* 21 (1992), 103–110.

Sansolo, Michael, "Going Green: Three Ways to Build Trust," *Progressive Grocer* (February 1991) 45–50.

Vandermerwe, Sandra, and Michael D. Oliff, "Customers Drive Corporations Green," *Long Range Planning* 23 (November-December 1990), 10–16.

Varadarajan, P. Rajan, "Marketing's Contribution to the Strategy Dialogue: The View from a Different Looking Glass," *Journal of the Academy of Marketing Science* 20 (Fall 1992), 335–344.

–5–

MEETING THE SUPERVALUE CHALLENGE

Philip Kotler

Philip Kotler is the S. C. Johnson & Son Distinguished Professor of International Marketing at Northwestern University's J.L. Kellogg Graduate School of Management. He is the author of more than 100 articles and 15 books, including *Marketing Management; Strategic Marketing for Nonprofit Organizations; Social Marketing; Marketing Places; Marketing Models;* and *The New Competition.* He has been a consultant to such companies as IBM, General Electric, AT&T, Bank of America, Merck, Motorola, Ford, and others. He holds honorary degrees from the University of Zurich and DePaul University, and has been a director and board of advisors' member of the American Marketing Association, Marketing Science Institute, The Drucker Foundation, Gemini, and The School of the Art Institute of Chicago. He received his M.A. from the University of Chicago and his Ph.D. from Massachusetts Institute of Technology, both in economics.

Futurescope

In the 1970s, consumers were ready to pay "more for more," and luxury goods flourished. In the 1980s, consumers began to demand "more for the same," and the discounting era grew strong. Today's consumers are now demanding "more for less," and the winners will be the supervalue marketers.

One of America's leading businessmen, Jack Welch of General Electric, recently observed: "The value decade is upon us. If you can't sell a top-quality product at the world's lowest price, you're going to be out of the game."

Translated, he is saying that companies must learn how to master high differentiation and low cost at the came time. This goes against Michael Porter's argument that the two disciplines are incompatible. High differentiation calls for investing in value-adding features that will unavoidably raise costs. Achieving low cost, on the other hand, called for mercilessly cutting costs to the bare bone.

Supervalue Companies

Yet some of today's most successful companies have mastered both disciplines. These companies have learned to produce supervalue. Among them are Dell Computer, Lexus, and Wal-Mart.

Dell Computer

As personal computers began to move into the commodity stage, Michael Dell, then 24 years of age, decided that people were ready to buy their computers through the mail. He believed that a mail-order vendor could offer both lower prices and better service than could computer store retailers. The key is to train highly competent consultants who are reachable by phone 24 hours a day. Retailers were often deficient in competent staff, and many closed their doors at 6:00 p.m. Dell achieved a phenomenal growth rate and led the personal computer industry in overall customer satisfaction.

Lexus

Toyota launched its high-end car, the Lexus, with the challenging headline: "Perhaps the First Time in History That Trading a $72,000 Car for a $36,000 Car Could Be Considered Trading Up." Not only did the car offer more quality per dollar, but also the whole selling philosophy was superior. Lexus spent as much time designing its dealerships as the car. Its showrooms are physically attractive. The customer enters and is offered coffee by the receptionist. The salesperson shows the cars, gives a generous test drive, and also gives a tour of the service bays. The interaction with the salesperson is cordial and professional, with the salesperson supplying accurate technical information. If the customer decides to buy the car, there is no haggling over price.

Wal-Mart

Wal-Mart's phenomenal growth into the country's largest retailer comes as no surprise, considering the supervalue that it generates. Two signs in huge letters appear in the front of every Wal-Mart store: "Everyday low prices" and "Customer Satisfaction Guaranteed." The shopper enters and is greeted by a friendly Wal-Mart employee who offers to help in any way. The shopper confronts a wide and deep assortment of nationally branded goods at very low prices. And the service is immediate and superior to that offered by many upscale department stores.

Rising to Supervalue Status

A number of other companies are working hard to provide supervalue to their target customers, including Hewlett-Packard, Home Depot, and American Airlines. These companies recognize that consumers are more educated and more able to recognize true customer value. Consumers are less taken in by designer labels and fancy frills. They want to deal with manufacturers and retailers who guarantee and deliver good value and who keep down their costs.

Section II
Creative Communications

The need to create messages that communicate effectively and persuasively with your customer has never been greater. Whether produced for a mass audience or for the emerging one-on-one marketing environment, these messages must function in the turbulent atmosphere of changing customer demands, a dynamic marketing environment, and changing organizational needs.

In "Creativity in Marketing," Arthur VanGundy identifies the principles of creativity necessary to meet the changing and sometimes conflicting needs of today's marketing organization, and in "Brainwriting: What to Do When There's Not a Cloud in the Brainstorming Sky," Greg Goodman does a whimsical yet serious exposition of new, no-risk ways to generate new ideas. In "The Future of Positioning," Jack Trout and Al Ries explore the problems of the "overcommunicated society" and its implications of ever-increasing noise in the global marketplace. The importance of positioning one's product properly in the mind of the consumer—and the challenges of doing so—will be greater than ever.

Public relations will play an especially important role in product positioning, according to Harold Bergen, in "The New Role of Public Relations in Marketing," as the significance of brands and generics shifts and the number of channels for reaching potential customers increases. But in an increasingly complex world the best-conceived marketing plans can go awry, and when they do a plan is essential to avoiding total calamity. Alan Leahigh gives prescriptions for handling adversity in "Crisis Management: Getting It Right When 'Things' Go Wrong."

On another level Shaun P. Gilmore and Cecil C. Hoge, Sr., explore how new technologies will impact communication with the customer. Gilmore analyzes the new dimensions of a now-familiar technology in "800 Service: The Next 25 Years" and the radical new future that awaits companies and customers alike. In "Electronic Marketing 2000" Hoge surveys the many new forms of electronic marketing that will soon be fixtures in the marketplace.

—6—

CREATIVITY IN MARKETING

Arthur B. VanGundy

Arthur B. VanGundy, Ph.D., is Professor of Communications at the University of Oklahoma, owner of the consulting firm VanGundy & Associates, Inc., and an associate of New Product Resources, Inc. He has written nine books on creativity and problem solving and has spoken at numerous conferences and professional meetings in the United States and abroad. VanGundy's consulting clients have included Carrier Corporation, Xerox, Monsanto, Kerr-McGee Chemical, AirCanada, McNeil Consumer Products (the "Tylenol" people), Eveready Battery, The American Chemical Society, Hallmark Cards, Mitsubishi Heavy Industries America, Hershey Foods, S.C. Johnson & Sons Company (Johnson Wax), Wisconsin Gas, Wyeth-Ayerst Pharmaceutical, the Singapore Civil Service Institute, and the Singapore Institute of Standards and Industrial Research. VanGundy holds a B.A. in psychology, an M.S. in personnel psychology, and a Ph.D. in education.

Organizations constantly must reinvent themselves while trying to maintain a degree of internal stability. It is not an easy job. Moreover, marketing is somewhat of a double-edged sword. Marketers might try to anticipate consumer desires, but consumers do not always know what they want. The telephone, for instance, was not instantly well-received. Letters and the telegraph had sufficed for years, so why change?

Although consumer desires are difficult to anticipate, marketers frequently excel at getting their messages across to consumers. Even if they don't know why it works, they do it successfully nonetheless. What effective marketers do is challenge assumptions and generate creative ways of attracting consumers' attention. Both of these behaviors represent primarily creative thinking skills. Unfortunately, many marketers do not know they have these skills or they tend to overlook potential contributions of creativity in general. Creativity and the creative problem-solving process have a lot to offer the marketing field. Unfortunately, creativity has gotten some bad press. (Perhaps it needs to be marketed better.)

Creativity is not some magical or mystical concept bestowed by the muses upon a few fortunate individuals. It is not unique only to artists. There are many different forms of creativity. Artistic creativity is one type, and marketing creativity is another. And it is not just a simple matter of "either you have it or you don't." It is something we all possess to one degree or another. Creativity is the ability to test assumptions, to see things from different perspectives, and to generate novel and useful ideas. If you can do these things, even moderately well, then you are creative.

If applied appropriately, creativity can define and sharpen your marketing strategy. It can help you to rethink your strategy to achieve, maintain, or improve competitive advantage. And it can assist you in exploiting potential marketing opportunities (Bobrow and Shafer, 1987). Creativity can be used to move: (1) existing products to existing markets (e.g., generate product improvements, new uses, marketing support), (2) existing products to new markets (e.g., generate new seg-

---

Futurescope

Marketing is a rather turbulent business. It is characterized by changing consumer demographics and a vast array of uncertainties, ranging from changing government regulations and technological advances to unclear interfaces with R&D and variable production cycles. These uncertainties and the rapid pace of change create new challenges for marketers. What worked in the past might no longer be effective. New creative strategies and philosophies are needed just to remain competitive.

ments and creative distribution channels), (3) new products to existing markets (e.g., generate special incentive programs and innovative marketing campaigns), and (4) new products to new markets (e.g., generate creative ways to offset the risks involved).

But wait. There's more! Creative also can help with the product mix (new ideas for planning, development, size, color, packaging, labeling), distribution mix (innovative ways to improve channels and activities, flows, inventory, handling, storage, transportation), the promotion mix (unique angles for advertising, sales, promotion, public relations, merchandising), and the pricing mix (creative ways to establish value to the customer). In short, creativity is an essential ingredient of the strategic marketing mix. Depending on how much risk is involved and how competitive the environment is, creative can even make the difference between marketing success and failure.

So, if creativity can help you, how can you get it and make it work for you? Well, you probably cannot "get it," any more than you suddenly can "get" intelligence or a different personality. And, if you work in an organization that is not supportive of new ideas, it will be more difficult to express your creativity. You can follow a few basic principles, however, and use some techniques to structure the creative idea-generation process.

Creativity Principles

There are many creativity principles, all of which can help you enhance your creative potential. Two principles, however, are more important than the others: (1) test all assumptions and (2) defer judgment while generating ideas.

Test Assumptions

Master escape artist Harry Houdini once was challenged by some small-town jailers to demonstrate his skills. Houdini was laced into a straitjacket, handcuffed, and placed in a jail cell. He quickly removed the straitjacket and handcuffs. Try as he might, however, he was unable to pick the lock to the cell door. He finally gave up and, in desperation, leaned against the cell door. As he did, he promptly fell onto the floor as the door swung open easily. You see, the jailers had neglected to lock the door. Houdini had failed to test the assumption that the door was locked!

A simple exercise I use in my seminars also illustrates the importance of testing assumptions: Draw a circle and pretend it is a pie. Now, cut the pie into eight pieces using three or fewer cuts. Go ahead. Give it a try. You will find that it is easy to get six or seven pieces. But your probably cannot get eight pieces unless you test assumptions. For instance, does the problem require the pie to be cut into equal sized pieces? Does it require pie-shaped pieces? Does it even require straight-line cuts? Does it specify the cutting instrument? The answer to all these questions, obviously, is no. The problem, however, can be solved only by asking these and similar questions. [Possible solutions: (1) Cut the pie into quarters and then draw a circle in the middle of the pie. (2) Cut the pie in half, stack it, cut the stack in half, stack all the pieces, and then cut that stack in half. (3) Design a seven-bladed knife with the blades radiating out, perpendicular to the handle. One stamp and you have eight pieces!]

Successful marketers have this ability to analyze a problem and recognize what information actually exists and what they are adding unnecessarily. If you make decisions based on nonexistent information, you will make your job a lot more difficult. As the cartoon character Pogo once said, "We have met the enemy and he is us."

One of my clients, an international air carrier, once assumed that their priority problem was devising ways to attract more customers. Their primary market was so competitive that all traditional marketing methods failed. However, once they generated data about the problem and produced new perspectives, they were able to test assumptions and redefine their strategy. For instance, their analyses revealed repeated concerns about prices, service, and comfort. After reviewing all the data, it appeared that their real problem was customer satisfaction. If they could satisfy current customers, they they could increase repeat business and attract new customers. Marketers cannot afford *not* to test and challenge assumptions. Survival and growth depend on this ability.

Defer Judgment

The second most important creativity principle is to defer judgment while generating ideas. Brainstorming pioneer Alex Osborn popularized this principle. And he was right. Numerous research studies have backed him up. You will get more ideas if you separate idea generation and evaluation. And, quite often, idea quantity breeds idea quality. Besides, a constant atmosphere of negative thinking can repress creative thoughts.

I once observed some marketing and advertising people brainstorm ideas for a promotional campaign to reintroduce an old product to a new market. After nearly every idea was proposed, someone would cite statistics and ask for supporting data and demographics. Needless to say, this session resulted in few ideas. Analysis paralysis prevailed once again. Compare this experience with a group I observed that deferred judgment while generating ideas. They used a variety of methods to think of a new food product for an existing market. Deferring judgment and using a variety of methods helped them to think of hundreds of ideas in a few hours. They then began reviewing their ideas and thought of even more new ones.

Every idea proposed in a group has value—no matter how silly or impractical it might seem at first. Even if it is not apparent how an idea might be used as a solution, it might stimulate someone else to think of a new idea. Ideas can help prompt other ideas. When generating ideas, remember this: Ideas are the raw material of solutions. When first proposed, an idea is a fragile creature that must be nourished and developed. Give new ideas a chance to become great ideas.

The Ideal Brainstorming Group

A relatively small percentage of the population seems to have a natural ability to generate ideas. If you belong to this group, then you do not need any help. Most of us, however, can benefit from ways to structure the idea-generation process. Before looking at idea-generation techniques, however, it is important to consider how to design a group for maximum brainstorming effectiveness. Although it also is possible to generate ideas individually, you will get more ideas from a group.

After reading the research literature, conducting research, and facilitating groups for almost 20 years, I have developed a few guidelines on how to put together the ideal brainstorming group. In no particular order, the guidelines are as follows:

1. Limit group size to no more than five or six people.

2. At a minimum, establish the ground rule of separating idea generation from idea evaluation.

3. Include a mixture of personality types in each group.

4. Use a variety of idea-generation methods, including those in which ideas are generated silently (so-called "brainwriting" methods).

5. Encourage a fun and playful atmosphere. Research has shown that groups in which humor is evident generate more ideas.

6. If possible, include one or two facilitators in each group. These individuals should be natural idea generators and have the ability to model and use many idea-generation approaches.

7. Keep the pace moving. When a group "dries up," move on to another technique. Setting goals and time limits also can spur idea productivity.

Most of the research literature shows that, all things being equal, a nominal brainwriting group will generate more ideas than a typical brainstorming group. That is, a "group" of four or five people who write down their ideas silently and then pool the result will produce more ideas (after eliminating duplicates) than another group of similar people who spend the same amount of time brainstorming. For one thing, nominal groups help ensure equal participation by eliminating conflicts and dominant personalities. Also, only one person can talk at a time in brainstorming groups, so nominal groups are more likely to list more ideas.

To compare different idea-generation methods, we recently conducted a research project at the University of Oklahoma (VanGundy, et al., in progress). We found that having group members write down their ideas and then pass them to other group members (to use for stimulation) was the best way to increase idea quantity. These interacting brainwriting groups generated significantly more ideas (an average of 121 ideas for 45 minutes) than both traditional nominal brainwriting groups (an average of 47 ideas) or brainstorming groups (an average of 30 ideas).

Do not interpret these results to mean that you should abandon traditional brainstorming. Brainstorming groups satisfy many social interaction needs that cannot be found in brainwriting groups. For this reason, I recommend always using a combination of brainwriting and brainstorming methods.

Idea-Generation Techniques

Most individuals and groups can use some help in generating ideas. Elsewhere I have described and evaluated the almost 100 creativity methods available (Van-Gundy, 1988, 1992). To illustrate how these methods can be used, I will briefly describe a few and provide examples using a problem from the product mix of marketing strategy: developing a new type of sock.

Pin Cards

This approach represents interacting brainwriting and originally was developed by Geschka, Schaude, and Schlicksupp (1973). Group members are given a stack of index cards and told to write down one idea on a card and pass it to the person on their right. This person examines the new idea and uses it to prompt additional ideas. They write down any new ideas (on a separate card) and pass all cards to the person on their right. This process continues until time is called (usually about 15–20 minutes). All of the idea cards are collected and then saved for later evaluation or sorted into idea categories or functional areas.

For instance, Greg might write down the idea of a sock with pictures of famous people on them. He then passes this idea card to Maria, who uses it to suggest socks with pictures of famous locations. She writes down this idea and passes the card to Chris, who uses it to suggest socks with holographic designs. All the while, any group member can write down and pass around any ideas they might think of.

Picture Stimulation

Geschka et al at the Battelle Institute in Frankfurt, Germany, developed different variations of this method. The basic procedure involves a group looking at a picture projected on a screen or flipping through specially constructed notebooks of pictures. The group selects a picture that is unrelated to the problem and describes it in detail. Next, they use their descriptions to help prompt ideas.

Suppose a group selects a picture of an old-fashioned mill located by a stream. They might write down some descriptions, such as: the mill is near water, there is running water, the water wheel turns with the water flow, the turning wheel grinds grain, there is an attached storage building, the water exerts pressure against the wheel, the faster the water flows, the faster the wheel turns. The group then examines each descriptor and tries to use it to stimulate ideas. In this case, they might think of the following ideas: (1) water-weighted socks for exercising (from "running water"), (2) small, built-in storage pouches (from "attached storage building"), (3) waterproof socks (from "mill near water"), and (4) the more the socks are pulled up, the better they fit (from "the faster the water flows, the faster the wheel turns").

Product Improvement CheckList (PICL)

VanGundy (1985) developed the Product Improvement CheckList as a brainstorming aid for both individuals and groups. It consists of a poster-sized worksheet printed on two sides with 576 stimulus words organized into four categories: Try To, Make It, Think Of, and Take Away or Add. For instance, Try To: slice it, sketch it, punch it, brush it, saturate it; Make It: transparent, portable, stretch, reflect, magnetic; Think Of: escalators, radios, time bombs, eggshells, boat rudders; Take Away or Add: traction, friction, zippers, movement, anticipation. There are several ways to use these random stimulus words to generate ideas. The simplest way is to select a word at random, see what ideas it stimulates, write them down, and then move on to another word.

Here are some sock ideas generated using PICL: (1) pump-up socks, like pump-up shoes (from "Try to punch it"); (2) perfume-scented socks (from "Try to saturate it"); (3) socks that expand into leggings (from "Try to stretch it"); (4) socks with mirrors or reflective material on them (from "Make it reflect"); (5) socks with interchangeable jewelry attached with magnets (from "Make it magnetic"); (6) cushion the bottom of socks with foam cells (from "Think of eggshells"); (7) rubber socks that (with attachments) can double as swimming flippers (from "Think of boat rudders"); (8) add zippers as a novelty for long socks (from "Take Away or Add zippers"); and (9) vibrating massage socks (from "Take Away or Add movement").

Semantic Intuition

The typical invention process involves inventing a product and then giving it a name. Schaude developed this technique by reversing the invention process: generating names and then using them to suggest product ideas. There are three basic steps involved.

1. Generate two lists of words associated with the problem area.

2. Randomly select one word from each list.

3. Use the word combinations to suggest ideas.

For instance, you might set up the sock problem by listing things associated with socks and people who wear socks (see Table 1).

Next, select words from each column and use them to generate ideas. Thus, you might think of the following ideas:(1) install cooling agents in the socks (from

Table 1

Socks	People Who Wear Socks
hot	walking
colors	washing
heel	running
material	darning
patterns	folding
moisture	pulling up
tightness	worn toes

"hot-walking"), (2) make the sock colors change after each washing (from "colors-washing"), (3) make the sock design patterns change as the socks are raised or lowered (from "patterns-pulling up"), or (4) put chemicals in the socks to absorb moisture during athletic activities (from "moisture-running").

The Bottom Line

If you test assumptions and use a variety of idea-generation methods, you can improve your strategic marketing performance. It might take a while, but the influx of new thinking and new ideas eventually will pay off. However, doing these things will not be enough. The bottom line is that creativity cannot flourish if it does not exist in a supportive environment. Several other ingredients also must exist for effective marketing creativity.

First, there must be top management support for new ways of doing things. This support must be translated into providing required resources as well as inspirational and psychological support. Second, the marketing department, like the organization itself, must develop a vision. In this case, the vision will be one of optimal marketing performance. This vision should be congruent with the organizational vision and refer to creative, innovative activities. As part of this vision, marketers must decide on their goals and core values. What are the essential marketing segments you want to serve? What is your niche? Who are your customers? How are you going to service them? Finally, the marketing vision must be articulated clearly to all relevant employees, with the joint goals of psychological and structural alignment. That is, employees must buy in to the vision (psychological alignment), and the mechanisms (e.g., regular idea-generation sessions) must be created or improved on to ensure creative thinking can flourish (structural alignment). To paraphrase Charles Kettering, you can be more creative, but you never will be if the only view you have is from the bottom of a rut.

References

Bobrow, E. E., and D. W. Shafer. *Pioneering New Products: A Market Survival Guide.* Homewood, Ill.: Dow Jones-Irwin, 1987.

Diehl, M., and W. Stroebe, "Productivity Loss in Idea-Generating Groups: Tracking Down the Blocking Effect, *Journal of Personality and Social Psychology 61* (3) (1991), 392–403.

Geschka, H., G. R. Schaude, and H. Schlicksupp, "Modern Techniques for Solving Problems," *Chemical Engineering* (August 1973), 91–97.

Isen, A. M., K. A. Daubman, and G. P. Nowicki, "Positive Affect Facilitates Creative Problem Solving," *Journal of Personality and Social Psychology 52* (6) (1987), 1127–1131.

Osborn, A. F. *Applied Imagination: Principles and Procedures of Creative Thinking,* 2nd ed. New York: Scribner's, 1957.

Schaude, G. R., "Methods of Idea Generation," in S. S. Gryskiewicz, ed, *Proceedings of Creativity Week I, 1978.* Greensboro, NC: The Center for Creative Leadership, 1979.

VanGundy, A. B. *The Product Improvement CheckList (PICL).* Norman, Okla.: VanGundy & Associates, 1985.

VanGundy, A. B. *Techniques of Structured Problem Solving,* 2nd ed. New York: Van Nostrand Reinhold Co., 1988.

VanGundy, A. B. *Idea Power: Techniques and Resources for Unleashing the Creativity in Your Organization.* New York: AMACOM, 1992.

VanGundy, A. B. *Brain Boosters: 100 Ways to Get Ideas and Beat the Competition.* New York: AMACOM, in progress.

Van Gundy, A. B., D. Hall, M. Myers, S. Moore, R. Clarke, M. Fairly, and A. Aw, "Overcoming Productivity Loss in Brainstorming and Brainwriting Groups," in progress.

Wizenberg, L., *The New Products Handbook.* Homewood, Ill.: Dow Jones-Irwin, 1986.

—7—
BRAINWRITING
What to Do When There's Not a Cloud in the Brainstorming Sky

Greg Goodman

Greg Goodman, Ed.D., is Process Manager of the All-Employee Systems Division of Maritz, Inc., a performance improvement firm based in Fenton, Missouri. Since joining Maritz, Goodman has worked with such clients as Siemens Medical Systems, IDS, General American Life, McDonald's, AT&T, Mallinckrodt Medical, General Electric, Ameritech, Georgia-Pacific, Transamerica, Bristol Meyers-Squibb, Baylor Medical Center, Monsanto, General Motors, and Fort Sanders Health System. He holds a doctorate degree in education from the University of Massachusetts-Amherst; an M.A. in biomedical communications from The Ohio State University; and a B.S., summa cum laude, in broadcasting, also from The Ohio State University.

You've been in this meeting, way too many times. There's a problem, and the boss uses the "B" word: "Let's brainstorm!"

Let's not, and say we did.

Don't get us wrong, brainstorming can be very productive. All you have to do is: remove the politics, make individuals feel they can't hide in the group, provide toys and music, muzzle the boss, and surgically remove every evaluative bone in every body.

Or, you can opt for brainwriting. The word *brainwriting* may conjure up images of dipping craniums in ink. That approach to brainwriting is optional and messy, but it's a great metaphor and potentially a great teambuilding activity.

Thinking under a Cloudless Sky

Brainwriting is brainstorming in silence and on paper. If used properly, brainwriting can deftly sidestep the bull associated with brainstorming.

Now, you could learn more about brainwriting by merely reading the rest of this article. You will, however, get better business results if you "do" a brainwriting action learning cycle.

Pick a problem—a real one. A problem whose solution you would be proud to tell the boss. Call a 30-minute meeting of five to seven people. Make sure you have the following combination of people: Some you respect, some you don't respect, some smart, some who think they are, some creative, some "others" (everyone is creative).

Follow these brainwriting steps: don't talk. Just write!

1. Following the brainstorming rules (these, or yours):

   - Don't criticize or judge

   - Go for quantity

   - Build from each other's ideas

   - Don't censor yourself

> ### Futurescope
> Ideas are the lifeblood of every organization, and good ones are the most difficult "commodity" to come by. A new technique called Brainwriting, built on the premises of Brainstorming, promises to be the way that successful organizations of the future will generate the quantity and quality of ideas needed for success.

2. Know what the problem is (not always as simple as it sounds). The key is common understanding.

3. Start with a blank form. Figure 1 is the form used in the Targeted Innovation program from the Center for Creative Leadership. Keeping the problem in mind, write three ideas across row one.

4. Then, trade for someone else's form from a pile in the middle of the table. Write three more ideas in row two. Use more of your own ideas or get them from ideas other people have written in previous rows.

5. Keep trading and filling in rows until the "popcorn stops popping."

6. Wait 30 to 60 seconds, then write one to three more ideas.

7. Say the following, "Time is up. You absolutely, positively can't write any more ideas." Then allow another 1 to 2 minutes for writing ideas.

Steps 1-5 are the basic building blocks of brainwriting. Steps 6 and 7 add more fun, get you more ideas, and appeal to paradigm punishers.

Don't be surprised if you get 150 to 200 ideas. Typically, solutions generated in brainwriting are not radical, but they are clever. Don't forget to thank everyone!

No Risk—in Any Setting

We hope you realize that brainwriting is not a risky proposition. In fact, we encourage you to repeat this highly productive process in the comfort of your own home, office, factory, ready room, nursing station, or favorite watering hole. The brainwriting technique is super, but phone booths are not recommended. Now that you've done it in one format, here are some more.

1. Good Graffiti:

- Get some of your kid's butcher-block paper, a really big piece.

- Write the problem statement on it. If your sense of cosmic correctness tells you to, write it at the top.

- Post the list in an accessible place. Behind your desk chair is not what we have in mind.

- Wait as long as you can stand it. Then wait a little longer to collect the voice of the people.

- Post a thank-you notice in said place. Add "Look for future idea challenges at a water cooler near you!"

Figure 1 Brainwriting

11	12	13
21	22	23
31	32	33
41	42	43
51	52	53
61	62	63
71	72	73

Adapted from a form attributed to Bernd Rohrbach. Rohrbach's form appeared in print in Johansson, B., *Kreativitat and Marketing*. H. Kern AG: Switzerland, 1978. © 1989, Center for Creative Leadership

2. You're a Card, Andy!

- Use one index card per idea in a group of five to seven people.

- Give everyone seven blank index cards as their starting "hand."

- Have people deal an idea card to whomever they wish after writing one idea on one card.

- When energy lulls, have everyone show their "hand."

- Create a "pot" of additional ideas, asking each person in turn to ante-up.

- The last person with an additional idea wins a date with the Trumps.

- It's then helpful to pin up all the cards in topical clusters for participant review.

- Participants then add cards to the clusters if more ideas are prompted from viewing the pin-ups.

3. McMurphy's Challenge. McMurphy's Challenge differs from previous techniques in that:

- Rather than a problem statement, the "thing" in the box is stated as a challenge rather than a problem because Toni McMurphy believes that positive thinking leads to increased creativity. We agree.

Figure 2: McMurphy's Challenge

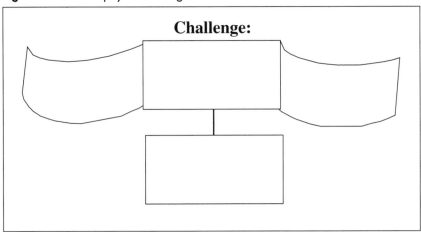

- Toni's form (Figure 2) allows for brainwriting around themes or strands of thought rather than totally random thinking.

Follow the five to seven brainwriting steps listed previously for best results. We find Toni's method particularly fruitful when previous thinking has identified "hot" strands of thought that are felt to be paths to idea "hits." And believe us, the hits will just keep on coming if you use brainwriting.

More Ways—More Sources

Now that you've lost your amateur status, let's give you some factoids about brainwriting before pressing on.

A lot of what we know about brainwriting comes from the research work of the Battelle Institute in Frankfurt, Germany, starting in 1971. Their American counterpart, the Center for Creative Leadership, has also greatly added to our knowledge since 1978.

People in the creativity biz may give you the "odd duck" stare if you use the brainwriting titles from this article. So, we'll translate them into academic for you:

- The "no-name" technique you first did is a variation of the 6-3-5 method called "Brainwriting Pool." That's why we had you jump right in rather than giving you a history lesson.

- Good Graffiti is a Gallery Method. You can give more structure to this method by having people work in separate rooms, break for a view in each other's "gallery," then go back to work in your own gallery incorporating ideas you found stimulating during your tour.

- You're a Card, Andy! is a Pin Card technique. Idea cards can also be passed around or left on the table for easy access while participants are generating ideas.

- McMurphy's Challenge can be used as a Brainwriting Pool or Gallery Method.

There are more psychologically-challenging brainwriting techniques on the market if you want to expand your repertoire. We suggest you get to know the resources listed in the reference section of this article.

Let us leave you now with two thoughts:

- Brainwriting encourages Trigger thinking—using one thought to trigger many thoughts. The more you use brainwriting and other creative problem solving techniques in your daily life, the more automatic trigger thinking becomes.

- And, most importantly: "To be truly creative, you must truly be free." Tensin Gyato, the thirteenth Dalai Lama.

Happy Trails.

For Further Reading

1. Center for Creative Leadership. Greensboro, NC.
2. Edward de Bono, *Lateral Thinking* (New York: Harper Colophon).
3. William C. Miller, *The Creative Edge* (New York: Addison-Wesley).
4. Arthur VanGundy, *Idea Power* (New York: AMACOM).

–8–

THE FUTURE OF POSITIONING

Jack Trout and Al Ries

Al Ries is chairman of Ries & Ries, a marketing strategy firm based in Great Neck, New York. Prior to establishing Ries & Ries, he was founder and chairman of the board of Trout & Ries, where he worked with Jack Trout for more than 26 years. Together, Trout and Ries have co-authored a number of industry classics and best-sellers, including *Positioning: The Battle for Your Mind; Marketing Warfare;* and *Bottom-Up Marketing.* Their latest book, *The 22 Immutable Laws of Marketing,* outlines the basic reasons marketing programs succeed or fail.

Jack Trout is president of Trout & Partners, a marketing strategy firm based in Greenwich, Connecticut. His clients include IBM, Burger King, Chase Manhattan, Xerox, Merck, Procter & Gamble, and other Fortune 500 companies. Trout was instrumental in developing the vital approach to marketing known as "positioning." Prior to forming his own consulting firm, Trout worked with General Electric and Uniroyal corporations, before joining Mr. Ries at Trout & Ries.

You might have heard the story about a traveler who asked a farmer for directions to a nearby town.

The farmer replied, "Well, you go down the road for a mile, turn left at the fork. No...that won't work. You turn around and drive for half a mile till you hit a stoplight, then turn right. No...that won't work either." After a long pause, the farmer looked at the confused traveler and said, "You know what, son, you can't get there from here!"

This happens also to be the spirit of positioning. You can spend millions of dollars on great advertising and still fail miserably if you don't play by the rules of a game called *positioning*. In other words, "You can't get there from here."

Today's marketplace is no longer responsive to strategies that worked in the past. There are just too many products, too many companies, and too much marketing noise. We have become an overcommunicated society.

If you have any doubts, just count the number of media that carry your communications. There is television (commercial, cable, and pay). There is radio (AM and FM). There is outdoor (posters, billboards, and spectaculars). There are newspapers. Direct mail. Mass Magazines. Class magazines. Enthusiast magazines. Business magazines. Trade magazines. Annuals. Semi-annuals. And, of course, buses, subways, and taxicabs. Generally speaking, anything that moves is usually carrying a "message from our sponsor."

The per-capita consumption of advertising in the United States is more than $400 per year. Thousands of messages compete daily for a share of the prospect's mind. And, make no mistake about it, the mind is the battleground.

To better understand what your message is up against, consider the mind as a memory bank of a computer. Like a memory bank, the mind has a slot or "position" for each bit of information it has chosen to retain. In operation, the mind is a lot like a computer.

But there is one important difference. A computer has to accept what is put into it. The human mind does not. In fact, it's quite the opposite. The mind, as a defense mechanism against the volume of today's communications, screens and rejects much of the information offered it.

Futurescope

Positioning is needed more than ever in the marketplace of the 21st century. Marketing noise will increase exponentially with increasing exposure to new electronic marketing media, such as international computer networks, electronic mail, and hypertext. The opening and shifting of international business opportunities will create new challenges for the positioning game as well.

In general, people accept only new information that matches their prior knowledge or experience (the mind's previous pattern of slots or positions). They filter out everything else. And it doesn't make much difference how creatively the new information is presented.

Years ago, when General Electric was trying to get into the mainframe computer business, it told prospects its computers were better than IBM's. But nobody believed GE. That didn't fit what most people thought about IBM. You would accept new information on light bulbs from GE, but not on computers. This explains the difficulty that GE or any other company faces when it tries to take its established position into a totally new field.

The mainframe computer "position" in the minds of most people was filled by a company called "IBM." For a competitive computer manufacturer to obtain a favorable position in the prospect's mind, it must either dislodge IBM or somehow relate the company to IBM's position.

Yet, too many companies embark on marketing and communications programs as if the competitor's position did not exist. They advertise their products in a vacuum and are disappointed when their messages fail to get through.

Successful companies today play a came called *positioning*. They are aware not only of their own positions, but also of those of their competitors. They know when they can get there from here and when they can't. It wasn't always this difficult. A quick look at the history of the communications business might give you a better understanding of how we got to the positioning era.

After World War II, the communications business was in an era marked by what Rosser Reeves called the unique selling proposition (USP). Marketing people focused their attention on products and product features. In a lot of ways, these were the good old days, when the "better mousetrap" and some money to promote it were all you needed.

But technology started to rear its ugly head, and it became more and more difficult to establish that unique selling proposition. An avalanche of me-too products ended the product era. Your "better mousetrap" was quickly followed by three more just like it, all claiming to be better than yours. It was an era in which "new and improved" was the watchword for marketing products.

The next phase was the image era. Successful companies like Kodak and DuPont found that reputation or image was more important in selling a product than any specific product feature. In particular, the programs of the new-technology companies (Xerox, IBM, Sony) were spectacularly successful. Those of older, established companies were less successful.

The architect of the image era was David Ogilvy. As he said in his famous speech on the subject, "Every advertisement is a long-term investment in the image of a brand." And he proved the validity of his ideas with programs for Rolls-Royce, Hathaway Shirts, Schweppes, and other products.

Just as me-too products killed the product era, the me-too companies killed the image era. As every company tried to establish an image for itself, the noise level became so high that relatively few companies succeeded. And most of the ones that made it, did it primarily with spectacular technical achievements, not spectacular advertising (Xerox and the plain-paper copier, for example).

Today we are in the positioning era, an era that recognizes both the importance of product features and the company image, but more than anything else stresses the need to create a position in the prospect's mind.

Positioning is a game in which the competitor's image is just as important as your own—sometimes more important. The famous campaign, "Avis is only No. 2 in rental cars. So why go with us? We try harder," was a classic example of establishing a position against the leader.

In the positioning era, the name of your company or product is especially important. Take airlines, for example. As more route structures overlap, your name can be an anchor, no matter how much money you spend.

Take Eastern Airlines, for example. Eastern was among the first to "paint the planes" and "dress up the flight attendants" in an effort to improve its reputation. Its advertising was beautifully done by the country's largest advertising agency. "The Wings of Man" was the theme, with music by the London Philharmonic Orchestra. And Eastern wasn't bashful when it came to spending money.

For all that money, what did you think of Eastern? Where did you think they flew? Up and down the East Coast, to Boston, Washington, Miami, right? Well, they also flew to St. Louis, New Orleans, Acapulco, Los Angeles. But Eastern had a regional name, and the more it promoted "Eastern," the more they "couldn't get there from here." And, of course, they wound up in bankruptcy court.

A bad name is one thing, but even worse is a program without a name. That sounds like it could never happen, doesn't it? Well, it does when companies use initials instead of a name. And you see this happening quite often in today's marketing arena.

What companies like ACF, AMP, GAF, and TRW fail to realize is that initials have to stand for something. GE stands for General Electric. And everyone knows it. These companies were given their nicknames by their customers. This is why they are so valuable.

When a company gives itself a nickname, it doesn't work as well. When General Aniline & Film changed its name to GAF, all it caused was confusion. And confusion is something the mind rejects, making it impossible to establish a position.

To test this point, we performed an awareness study on a match sample of both "name" companies and "initial" companies. The survey was conducted over a *Business Week* subscriber list, and companies were selected that had corporate marketing programs running. The "name" companies had an average recognition score that was 19 percent higher than the average score of the "initial" companies.

The toughest marketing problems occur when a company competes with another company that has a strong, established position. For the best example, let's return to the ancient world of Snow White and the seven dwarfs. That is, the mainframe computer business when IBM was riding high with 70 percent of the market and 100 percent of the profits.

How do you advertise and market against this kind of overwhelming position? Well, first you have to recognize it. Then you don't do the thing that too many people in the computer field do—act like IBM. A company has no hope to make progress head-on against the position that IBM has established. And history has proved this to be true.

The small companies in the field recognized this. But the big companies thought they could take their strong positions against IBM. Well, as one disgruntled executive was overheard to say, "There just isn't enough money in the world." You can't get there from here. A better strategy for IBM's competitors would have been to take advantage of whatever positions they already own in their prospects' minds and relate them to a new position in computers.

General Electric was a leader in computer time-sharing. This could have been an especially appropriate move, because GE was one of the biggest users of computers. And time-sharing was a user-oriented idea.

RCA was a leader in communications. If it had positioned a computer line that related to its business in communications (a communications computer), it could have taken advantage of its own position. As it turned out, communications accounted for almost half of the computer market.

The point is that it's almost impossible to dislodge a strongly dug-in leader who owns the high ground. You're a lot better off to open up a new front or position—that is, unless you enjoy being shot up.

Applying Positioning to a Brand or Company

If you want to apply positioning thinking to a brand or a company, here are six questions to ask yourself.

What position, if any, do we already own in the prospect's mind? Get the answer to this question from the marketplace, not from the marketing manager. If this requires a few dollars for research, so be it. Spend the money.

What position do we want to own? Here is where you bring out your crystal ball and try to figure out the best position to own from a long-term point of view.

What companies must be outgunned if we are to establish that position? If your proposed position calls for a head-to-head approach against a market leader, forget it. It's better to go around an obstacle rather than over it. Back up. Try to select a position that no one else has a firm grip on.

Do we have enough marketing money to occupy and hold the position? The big obstacle to successful positioning is attempting to achieve the impossible. It takes money to build a share of mind. It takes money to establish a position. It takes money to hold a position once you've established it.

Do we have the guts to stick with one consistent positioning concept? With the noise level out there, a company has to be bold enough and consistent enough to cut through. The first step in a positioning program normally entails running fewer programs, but strong ones. The sound simple but actually runs counter to what usually happens as corporations get larger. They normally run more programs, but weaker ones. It's this fragmentation that can make many large advertising budgets just about invisible in today's media storm.

Does our creative approach match our positioning strategy? Creative people often resist positioning thinking, because they believe it restricts their creativity. And it does. But creativity isn't the objective of advertising in the year 2000. Even communications itself isn't the objective. The name of the marketing game is *positioning*. And only the better players will survive.

THE NEW ROLE OF PUBLIC RELATIONS IN MARKETING

Harold A. Bergen

Harold A. Bergen is Executive Vice President of Ruder-Finn, Chicago. He has served companies, associations, and governments in corporate, financial, marketing, employee, government, crisis management, and community relations programs. Before entering public relations, he was editor of *Industry and Power* magazine, senior associate editor of *Consulting Engineer* magazine, and manager of technical publications for the Raytheon Company. He is an active member of the Public Relations Society of America and has written and lectured extensively on public relations.

Compared with other forms of mass communication in which the media are paid (such as advertising), public relations offers these advantages:

- Much greater credibility that derives from the implied editorial endorsement of media or the implied approval of other third-party cooperating organizations

- Much less cost

On the other hand, paid media advertising offers total control of copy, art, positioning, and timing, as well as the opportunity to repeat the same messages in given media.

Publicity Basics

Traditionally, public relations focuses primarily on generating publicity in print and electronic media that reach end users as well as the influentials in the marketing channels that connect sources with users. The objective, at a minimum, is to strategically position the organization's name, products, services, or advocacies in a favorable and highly credible environment. The more ambitious objective is to move the audiences to buy and approve or to not interfere with action being advocated.

The target media for publicity campaigns must be as carefully selected as are media for paid advertising campaigns to avoid wasting time and money as well as to avoid antagonizing media whose support may be needed later.

Futurescope

Public relations can play a powerful and cost-effective role in marketing products, services, and concepts. And as the year 2000 approaches, that role will be played out in ever-altered modes as distribution channels change, as the significance of brands and generics shifts, and as communications channels for reaching end users proliferate. As much as cable television already has multiplied the opportunities for publicity, these will escalate as cable brings us in hundreds of channels, including many narrow-interest channels that can be especially important for particular marketing programs. Virtual reality, infomercials, home shopping networks, and interactive information networks also are reshaping the media landscape, as is database marketing. And technology is being developed to deliver newspapers electronically, with certain editorial material given priority based on the subscribers' expressed interests.

Publicity, then can be created for submission to trade, business, and professional media as well as to general consumer, special-interest, and politically oriented outlets. The scope of media within a public relations program can extend to direct mail, point-of-purchase materials, and public service announcements.

Media selection should follow from research into who affects the market (positively and negatively) for particular products, services, and concepts, and which media reach them most effectively and efficiently. In the case of pharmaceuticals, for example, doctors and pharmacists are much more influential than end users.

Then the target media must be studied to see what kinds of material they use, and in what formats: general news of people, organizations, and events; new products; new literature; research findings; feature articles (staff written or bylined by others); photo features; newsletter briefs; letters; editorials (staff written and/or guest authored); interviews (in person and call-in); or audio or video tapes.

A word of caution. Publicity for branded products and services is much harder to generate than for un-branded ones, because the editorial world looks on brand owners as partial, even biased. Associations and professional societies are looked on as much less biased and more independent authoritative sources—except those advocacy organizations that obviously exist to promote a point of view with respect to a contentious issue.

Creating Publicity

To take best advantage of the various formats available in the media, publicity must be created that emulates those formats and that satisfies the needs and interests of the media's audiences. Perennially, editors and broadcasters complain that they get huge amounts of material that is outside their formats or their audience interests. Some of the tried and true formats for publicity include news releases, features, tie-ins, success stories, spokesperson tours, created events, and teaching materials.

News Releases

Broadly distributed news releases create publicity by reporting on people, new products, new literature, crisis situations, research, awards, organizational plans, annual or special events, speeches, and organizational milestones. These generally are distributed widely to all potentially interested media.

News reported through releases about organizations as such helps build awareness and reputation for their products, services, or concepts. Especially in business-to-business marketing, the reputation of the organization can be as important as what it markets. And in the case of crisis, such as product tampering (remember Tylenol and Diet Pepsi), news about corporate performance certainly affects customer acceptance in the marketplace.

Distribution most often is by mail, sometimes backed up by fax, messenger, or paid newswire. (Back-up is a requirement for financial news defined as "material" by the Securities and Exchange Commission for publicly held corporations.) Video news releases (VNRs) are becoming more and more popular, although they are still very expensive on a cpm basis. VNRs are very cost-effective in instances of product recall, however, because of the very high usage rate generally achieved.

Features

Generated on a relatively restricted basis (often as "exclusives" or "exclusives in your field/area"), features are written either by media staff or outside authors. Features bylined by media staff generally report on trends and so are likely to be a bit more time sensitive, such as those on fashion, entertainment, sports, economics, and politics. Others can be anticipated, such as holiday specials or scheduled events. Some are more and less time sensitive, such as those on travel destinations, food products, real estate, and automotive.

Media that are fully staff written, such as *The Wall Street Journal* and *Business Week,* still can be approached with story ideas and interview suggestions that stimulate coverage of subjects that serve marketing purposes. The trick is to find the right editor/reporter/broadcaster and to come up with an approach they think will interest their audience.

Features written by outside authors are widely used by enthusiast, special-interest and trade media. They generally are accepted at face value but might be subject to a review by a jury of peers if they are professional papers (as for a technical journal). These features generally are less timely than fast-breaking news and often are on a how-to subject—how to buy, select, repair, budget, dress, choose, maintain, repair, make (e.g., recipes)—all somehow involving the product, service, or concept being marketed. They also might discuss trends, historical background, or personalities.

Of growing important in just about all media is the op-ed written by an outside author (usually a recognized authority) to advocate a viewpoint or action. From big-city metropolitan newspapers to the narrowest of niche market media, the op-ed is an increasingly available outlet to market a concept or advance a cause. This concept extends to radio and television, where talk show and editorial replay formats often are available.

Tie-ins

Another way to create publicity in print and electronic media is to create tie-ins and sponsorships with third parties. These could involve cause-oriented programs and events developed with nonprofit organizations concerned with health, environment, product safety, discrimination, fiscal responsibility, fund raising, or similar matters. Tie-ins also can be created with profit-making organizations: shopping malls, airlines, destinations, media or entertainment, and sports events. Or publicity-generating tie-ins can relate to events already created by others to generate publicity: parades, anniversaries, meetings, conferences, contests, and awards.

The most prevalent forms of tie-ins are offers of products or services as prizes and funding of awards, scholarships, and events—all in return for acknowledgments or visible participation.

Success Stories

Although bad news seems to be the staple of the editorial world, room is available for success stories about people and things. Business publications, in particular, welcome success stories that document how some change reduces costs or saves time. And personal achievements, especially in behalf of causes, can generate coverage. Success stories can be handled as widely distributed news releases or selectively targeted features, depending on the appeal and the nature of the media selected.

Spokesperson Tours

The most effective, but expensive, publicity generator is the spokesperson tour, by a publicist alone or with an organizational spokesperson. Meeting the media face to face is by far the most effective placement technique. Spokespersons can be corporate or elected leaders or authority figures in relevant fields. Editorial calls by spokespersons can be tied into their appearances at local or national meetings. (Avoid celebrities whose own personas will absorb all of the media's attention.) Expenses can be cut with satellite television tours, which are becoming increasingly popular.

Created Events

Events can be created to generate publicity in support of marketing. These include anniversary celebrations, community open houses, new facilities dedications, awards presentations, ground breakings, topping out ceremonies, convention opening ceremonies, hospitality suites, and mayoral or gubernatorial proclamation photo opportunities.

Teaching Materials

Educators at almost all grade levels welcome materials for classroom use that promote awareness of products, services, and concepts if the materials are educationally sound and not too commercial. Generic references are much more welcome than are brand name mentions. This means that material coming from associations generally will be more welcome.

Trends

Because media publicity is such a large part of most public relations programs, what affects media affects public relations opportunities. Some sources report a shift in marketing budgets from trade promotion to media advertising, which increases availability of space for publicity. The media continue to proliferate as consumer interests and technology expand, creating new publicity opportunities. Media serving these often can be more important than nationally circulated general interest media.

Merchandising

Publicity can have a very productive afterlife if merchandised. It can be repackaged as individual reprints or tapes for mailing to the target audiences. And it can be reformatted into newsletters. These materials also can be used at meetings and conventions, in annual reports, and in fund-raising programs. Some organization include reprints in response to requests for bids or in funds solicitation programs.

Programming

Programming for public relations support of marketing involves both scheduling and budgeting. Most programs can be coordinated with the total marketing effort to support it on a timely basis over a 12-month period and beyond. All schedules, especially for new product introductions, should take account of both preparation time and media lead times. for example, most major monthlies close their Christmas coverage by July 1. Note, too, that media deadlines are just that: the very last date at which something very important can be squeezed in.

Budgeting should be based on the total time cost (including benefits and overheads) of all the persons working on the program plus out-of-pocket expenses. Because public relations has an opportunistic dimension to it, provide an extra 5–10 percent as a contingency budget item to service the unexpected but worthwhile options that will surely come up.

Be generous when scheduling and budgeting. Underestimating the time it takes to do things is a common mistake. Creativity is not enough. Accountability is in, which means being on time, on target, and on budget is essential. With realistic planning and budgeting, public relations earns a respected place in marketing programs for products, services, and concepts.

–10–

CRISIS MANAGEMENT

Getting It Right When "Things" Go Wrong

Alan K. Leahigh

Alan K. Leahigh is Executive Vice President of Public Communications Inc., counselors in corporate, marketing, public affairs, financial, and institutional communications. A partner in the firm, he has more than 25 years of professional communications experience, and shares management responsibility for marketing, public affairs, health care, and general public relations accounts. He holds a bachelor of arts degree in political science from Illinois Wesleyan University, Bloomington, and a master of arts in journalism from the University of Missouri, Columbia.

You seem to have gotten it right. Your product launch was a success. Sales are running ahead of projections. Your product has an established image of quality and value.

Then it happens. A single telephone call and the bottom drops out. Now everything you've worked for depends on the decisions you make and the actions you take during the next several hours.

It may be a product-related crisis: a manufacturing error, a packaging mistake, a product tampering, a regulatory investigation, a class-action lawsuit, a boycott or protest by an activist group, the need for a recall.

Or the crisis might not be directly related to your product or service at all, but it nevertheless can disrupt your marketing and sales: a labor dispute, a plant closing, an industrial accident, a corporate acquisition or reorganization.

A single even can threaten to obliterate all the equity of past market development. Poorly handled, the crisis also can threaten future sales of your product or service. When the rug is pulled out, you want to be able to land on your feet. By planning ahead, you can be prepared for the unthinkable. Here is what you need to do:

- Assess your crisis vulnerabilities

- Develop a crisis prevention program

- Establish an early-warning system

- Prepare a crisis communications plan

- Learn some basic media relations skills

If you are part of a large firm or corporation, you probably have a public relations officer or department that has experience or training in managing crisis communications. You'll want to work closely with the public relations staff in anticipating and responding to crises.

The larger the crisis, the greater the media interest. Reporters will want to know the details of the crisis and how you are handling it. Your company probably has a policy that all contacts with the media must be coordinated through the public relations department. Your role might be one of providing information to the principal spokesperson, perhaps your company's chief executive officer.

Principles of Crisis Management

When confronting a public relations crisis related to your product or service, your actions can be guided by some bedrock principles. Here is a checklist:

1. **People come first.** Think and act in terms of the impact of the crisis on people: community, employees, neighbors, customers. People must always be placed ahead of product, profits, property, or politics.

2. **Tell the truth.** Accept the fact that the truth will come out. Deceptions, incomplete information, and half-truths invariably worsen a crisis and devastate your credibility when the truth later emerges.

3. **Get the best, most complete information.** To act effectively, you need to know as much as possible about the crisis and as quickly as possible. What happened? When did it happen? How did it happen? Who was involved? What is happening at the present time? What most likely will happen next?

4. **Create an inventory of what you don't know.** You might not be able to completely undo the damage, but there probably are steps you can take to help restore the situation and demonstrate your sincere concern about it.

5. **Decide your best remedy for the situation.** You might not be able to completely undo the damage, but there probably are steps you can take to help restore the situation and demonstrate your sincere concern about it.

6. **Identify the audiences.** Decide which people need information first. Who are the most affected? Give particular attention to internal audiences such as employees and their families.

7. **Release any bad news completely, clearly, and quickly.** News that is released in dribbles prolongs the crisis and causes everyone to wonder what is next and when the series of bad news will end.

There is an old saying: "Feed the bears or they'll eat you." If reporters don't obtain useful information from you, they will find it somewhere else. Establish your company as the primary source of information for the media. The sooner reporters recognize that your company is the best, fastest, and most complete source of information, the less likely it is that they will seek information from someone else. The more responsive and candid you are, the better your chance for fair, balanced, and accurate press treatment.

And the sooner reporters have the facts—both positive and negative—the quicker the story will cease to be newsworthy. Holding back information so as not

Futurescope

To address crisis management in the coming decades, it is necessary to begin now to anticipate your organization's vulnerabilities. The increasingly dangerous, unstable society of the 21st century means that organizations must strive more than ever to develop relationships of trust with their publics. The split-second reporting of tragic events presents new challenges for the crisis management team.

to alarm the public or employees is a disservice to those you are supposedly protecting. They will be alarmed much more when they find out you've held back information. If anyone suggests to you that information should be withheld in order to "reassure" or "not alarm" the public, a red flag should go up in your mind. It's a trap.

Checklist for Action

Based on the principles for crisis management outlined above, here is your checklist for action. Determine all of the following points:

1. **The main issue.** What will be of greatest concern to internal and external publics?

2. **Who is affected?** Those most affected should receive the first attention.

3. **Whether wrongdoing is implied.** Is the crisis the consequence of someone's error or omission? Is your company a victim or the perpetrator?

4. **Probable level of public interest.** Don't overreact or underreact. Your response should be commensurate with the interests of your audience.

5. **Your strengths in the matter.** What kind of public and community relations equity can you draw on to help you through the crisis?

6. **Steps that can correct or address the matter.** If possible, include in your first public statements about the crisis the steps you are taking, or plan to take, to correct the damage or offset its effects.

7. **Members of the crisis team.** Surround yourself with people who can help you gather and analyze information, develop communications strategy, and manage information dissemination.

8. **The spokesperson.** In times of crisis, the best spokespersons are either at the scene or at the top. Instruct staff and the telephone switchboard to refer all calls to the crisis team and its spokesperson.

9. **Methods of two-way communications.** Obviously you will want to use the best methods for disseminating information to key publics. But also determine the best ways to receive information from key publics. The inbound information will help you determine how well you are communicating and what else needs to be said or done.

Methods of Disclosure

You've assessed the crisis, gathered as much information as is immediately available, and decided on the initial remedies. It's now time to communicate. Usually this means a meeting with the media. How you disclose information about the crisis can often say as much about the situation and about your company as the actual content of your message.

- **Be compassionate.** Show by word and deeds that your overriding concern is the people adversely affected by the crisis.

- **Show you are in charge.** To earn public confidence, show that you are taking deliberate steps to address the crisis and bring about the best possible conclusion. Those around you may be bewildered, but you need to show that you can keep your head.

- **Keep it simple.** The crisis, its causes, and its ramifications might be complex and far-reaching, but probably there are a few key pieces of information that are of greatest public importance. Focus on those. Broadcast media, in particular, have difficulty managing more than two or three points. Help sort out the situation for your audience. If helpful, use photos or charts.

- **Express natural emotions.** This is not the time to appear cold and detached. The public will want to see that you are human and caring. Express your natural emotions. Are you horrified? Saddened? Dismayed? Your humanity and your honest concern are essential in communicating during a crisis.

- **Keep ahead of the release of information.** Show that you are the best source of accurate information. If media representatives find that they can obtain information faster or better elsewhere, you will lose control of the release of information.

- **Anticipate questions.** In whatever time is available before meeting the media, imagine the questions that you are likely to be asked. You might want an objective party to help you anticipate the questions. Determine the answers that you will give.

- **Don't speculate.** There might be questions about what will happen next and the consequences of the crisis. Provide only information of which you are certain. Don't guess about next steps and consequences. You will be embarrassed if later developments show that you guessed wrong.

- **If you are not sure, say so.** There might be information that is not yet available. Define the things that you do know and don't know. If possible, explain when you expect to have the missing information.

- **If you can't answer, explain why.** There might be some information that cannot be released. Give the reason the question cannot be answered.

- **Conduct rumor control.** Set up listening posts to snare misinformation. Don't let rumors build or fester. Deal with them immediately. Confirm them or deny them.

Crisis Audit

One of the best ways to sensitize yourself and your organization to potential crises is to conduct a crisis audit to determine your vulnerabilities.

Start by making a list of potential crises that would apply to your product and company. For example: product failure, product tampering, product recall, regulatory action, work stoppage, employee layoff, fire, explosion, collapse, terrorist attack, chemical leak, power outage, water cutoff, kidnapping, hostile takeover.

Talk to those who know what could happen—front-line managers, technical staff, outside sources—to discover potential trouble spots. Questions to ask include: Where are the greatest risks? What specifically could happen? How likely is it? How severe would the impact be? What groups would be affected? Look for worst-case scenarios.

Your crisis vulnerability audit should also include any industry-wide issues that might affect your product category or your company. As part of your plan, address the following points:

- Carefully anticipate the issues you might face. Together with management, develop an effective system for monitoring and anticipating public issues.
- Develop strategies and a plan for dealing with these issues in a manner consistent with overall corporate objectives.
- Decide on the protocol for managing communications about any industry-wide crisis that might touch on your product or company.
- Identify and analyze your key publics, including your own employees, customers, suppliers, government regulators, and elected officials.
- Determine how best to communicate with each key public.
- Designate a crisis control officer and a crisis team.
- Determine who will be spokesperson.
- Prepare comprehensive media lists, so you can initiate immediate contact with reporters when needed rather than simply react to media inquiries.
- Involve corporate management at all levels in understanding the issues. Give local plant managers the necessary training to successfully initiate issue management strategies at the community level.
- Permit properly trained managers to initiate proactive issues management programs.

Crisis Prevention

As always, a good offense is your best defense. How your company conducts its day-to-day business can determine the likelihood of your having to manage a crisis.

- Develop relationships of trust. If your customers, suppliers, employees, and others know that you are reputable and trustworthy, they will want to stand by you in a time of crisis.

- Be open, honest, and straightforward in all communications. Deceive your publics once, and they will always be skeptical about what you tell them.

- Anticipate problems and issues. One of the saddest comments is, "We should have seen the crisis brewing."

- Communicate aggressively. Don't let an emergency be the first time that anyone has ever heard from you. Low-profile companies can dodge some of the smaller issues, but they are in a deficit position when a big crisis occurs.

- Build coalitions with other groups. If you have good relations with customer organizations, industry associations, supplier organizations, government agencies, local officials, and civic groups, you can draw on those friendships in times of crisis.

In summary, establish a "good citizen" corporate image. Then when the crisis occurs—and sooner or later it will—your skilled management of the emergency and the store of consumer confidence will bring you through with intact credibility and intact markets.

−11−
800 SERVICE: THE NEXT 25 YEARS

Shaun P. Gilmore

Shaun P. Gilmore is Vice President of Global Consumer Communications Services for AT&T. He has held a variety of management positions at AT&T since first arriving at the firm in 1980, including both Operations Vice President of Inbound Services and Director of 800 Services Product Management and Marketing. He holds an M.B.A. in finance from Harvard Business School.

Since AT&T launched toll-free calling in 1967, 800 service has virtually revolutionized the way companies and consumers do business, nationwide and worldwide. In its 26-year history, toll-free calling has created whole new markets, enlarged existing ones, and made businesses more competitive at home and abroad.

A widely accepted way of promoting communications, an 800 number sends a clear message. Its owner-business is saying that customers or constituents are so important that it is willing to pay for the call, whether it be an order, a customer inquiry, a polling sample, or some other concern. The same is true of someone who has an 800 number at home.

As 800 service has grown internationally and even found its way into the home, so have its applications. No longer does 800 service simply handle collect sales calls; it has become a powerful tool for over-the-phone assistance and information. Although 49 percent of AT&T's business customers still use 800 service for sales and order-taking, 21 percent use the service for product and service inquiries, and 19 percent for internal applications. Another 12 percent use 800 service for credit card approvals, reservations, trouble reports, and consumer hotlines.

From its beginning as interstate INWARD WATS, used by a few large companies to receive collect calls from major customers and suppliers, 800 service has grown into a major industry in its own right. If AT&T's 800 service were a separate company, it would rank among the nation's top 250 businesses.

Today, some 40 percent of the 150 million calls carried on AT&T's long-distance network on an average business day are 800 calls. More than 11.72 billion 800 calls were made in 1992, the 25th year. History was made during the airline industry's promotions in June 1992, when long-distance calling reached an all-time

Futurescope

The 800 service industry is working hard to make the next 25 years of toll-free calling as revolutionary and valuable for business as the past quarter-century. The industry is developing new services that cater to the needs of its business customers and move beyond merely completing a call to completing an entire business transaction. In the next few years, a shopper seeking new shoes may call an 800 number and speak to a computer through a portable, pocket-sized phone. After asking for the latest selection of footwear, video pictures of the shoes are sent to the caller's videophone, or to a television at his or her home or in the office. The caller may purchase the shoes by simply asking for them—all without talking to a sales representative. Sound farfetched? Computers that recognize speech have been commercially available since the middle of the 1980s. Today, such systems typically recognize numbers from zero to nine, "yes," "no," and a dozen or so other words.

high on the AT&T network, and 800 calls for the first time surpassed the 50 percent level. American businesses currently handle 800 calls from more than 67 countries. More than half a million businesses and government agencies accept calls on more than 2.5 million 800 numbers, and those numbers are growing daily.

Evolution of 800 Service

As 800 service evolved, it went through three separate phases: automated collect calls, the worldwide intelligence network, and the electronic storefront.

Automated Collect Calls

In the automated collect call phase (1967–1976), 800 calling grew slowly. Created as a solution to an anticipated shortage of telephone company operators, 800 service was not part of a grand marketing vision. During this time, however, some entrepreneurial businesses began using 800 numbers in their television pitches to help sell inexpensive housewares, and 800 service quickly became associated with the products it helped sell. But other businesses, such as the Whirlpool Corporation, with an entrenched customer-service philosophy, saw hidden possibilities in the appeal of free calls for consumers. In 1967, Whirlpool's 800 number drew 10,000 toll-free calls, many from consumers curious to see what toll-free service was all about.

Worldwide Intelligence Network

The second phase of 800 calling's evolution, from 1977 to 1986, coincided with the coming of age of the AT&T worldwide intelligent network. Fueling the explosive growth of 800 service in the 70s and 80s was the installation of common channel signaling in AT&T's network, which made it possible to connect calls faster than ever. The creation of computerized databases in the network, a second powerful innovation, allowed businesses to advertise a single 800 number anywhere in the United States. The single nationwide number freed businesses from having different 800 numbers in different states.

These databases also allowed 800 calls to be routed to different offices or call centers based on the time of day, the day of the week, or the point of origination. These emerging capabilities helped businesses expand their markets and hours of service at a minimal cost.

As the popularity of toll-free calling increased, businesses awakened to the service and sales potential of single-number 800 service. National advertising began to routinely include 800 telephone numbers. Blue-chip corporations jumped on the 800 bandwagon. Start-up businesses learned of its power. Consumers, affluent baby boomers, and women entering the nation's work force discovered a fast, convenient way to shop and, in the process, helped spend the U.S. economy out of recession in the 70s.

Electronic Storefront

In the third phase of the service's evolution, from 1987 to the present, the electronic storefront unfolded. Carrier competition emerged. Changes in the regulation of telecommunications service charges brought prices down. And shrinking leisure time led consumers increasingly to shop by phone for time-saving products and services. According to a recent survey, American consumers, on the average, have made four 800 calls in the past three months, and over half of them have made a toll-free purchase during the same time. Annually 75 percent of American consumers make more than 17 calls to businesses that offer 800 numbers.

The Way America Shops

Small businesses enjoyed spectacular growth overnight as the popularity of catalog shopping increased sharply. Catalog sales rose an astonishing 93 percent between 1983 and 1989. Savvy marketers invented vanity 800 numbers: 1-800-FLOWERS, 1-800-4-CAVIAR, 1-800-451-JAVA, 1-800-HOLIDAY, 1-800-DEN-TIST, and 1-800-BYA-BOOT are a sampling.

To put all this in perspective, today the U.S. telemarketing industry employs 4 million people; spends $80–$90 billion a year on marketing, sales, and service; and generates more than $250 billion in sales, surpassing the gross domestic product of all but the 12 largest industrialized nations.

Even consumers are getting into the act, demanding 800 service for the home. Nowadays, people are using it as a convenient way to keep in touch with children away at college, family members who travel, and with relatives and friends.

And among major business customers, in 1992 Whirlpool, a corporate pioneer in toll-free calling for sales and service, answered 1.7 million consumer calls over its original 800 number—with a force of customer representatives 45 times larger than its staff 26 years ago.

Expanding its efforts to help its customers and consumers do business, AT&T offers nationwide toll-free directories with more than 150,000 listings. And people without directories can call 1-800-555-1212 for directory assistance on toll-free numbers.

Technologies to Reach
Rotary-Phone and Mobile Callers

Thanks to AT&T Speech Recognition, rotary-phone callers are no longer left on hold waiting for operators to redirect their calls. This technology allows businesses to reach new market segments at reduced costs. Rotary phones still account for as many as 30 percent of the residential phones in the United States and a much higher percentage abroad. Introduced in 1993, speech recognition allows such callers to give voice responses to interactive menus that forward their calls to the right department without the use of operators. Now, businesses may prompt callers to "SPEAK or PUSH one...if you want the sales department." The service is accurate more than 97 percent of the time, accommodating many different dialects and accents. Soon computers will recognize thousands of words in a variety of languages.

What does the future hold? A new technology under development by AT&T Bell Laboratories would please even Dick Tracy: an 800 number that follows you around no matter where you go, much like the new AT&T EasyReach℠ 700 Service. The receiver is not a wristwatch, but the idea is similar. A small, hand-held phone includes a device similar to a pager. When someone dials your personal 800 number, the signal is broadcast nationwide—or worldwide—and is picked up by the pager. Within a split second, the pager lets you know about the call and prompts your phone to call back and complete the connection.

Modern Wizardry: Complete Transactions

The use of voice response units is a harbinger of a new complete-the-transaction environment, the next phase in the evolution of 800 services. Already, the marriage of the telephone with computer databases helps marketers identify market segments for their products, provides potential customers with more complete information, and even ships products—while taking care of many bookkeeping functions as well. Much of this technology is commercially available now or quickly moving toward the marketplace.

Today, many people check their credit-card and bank-account balances over 800 lines without operator assistance, and more and more people use their touch-tone phones to transfer funds between accounts and to make purchases. For the past few years, customers of discount brokerages and financial services have been able to obtain their balances, hear the latest stock market information, and complete stock purchases from their touch-tone phone, 24 hours a day. Callers simply dial an 800 number, enter a personal identification number, and follow a series of spoken instructions. It has generated so many sales for one company that the 800 service has become, in effect, its largest "branch office."

Another new 800-based service enables callers to speak with a florist closest to the address where they want flowers delivered simply by entering the zip code. The long-distance network and computers do the rest. By contacting a local florist directly, callers can find out what flowers are fresh and available.

Small businesses are increasingly using such services as a cost-effective way to expand their markets. These technologies do not reside in the customer's office, but in the long-distance network. One such technology, called AT&T InfoWorx® is a network-based system that not only accepts 800 calls, but also can communicate with a variety of computers to send and retrieve information. In the case of the floral service, InfoWorx accepts the call, asks the caller questions, and finds the nearest florist from another computer with a list of zip codes. If that's not enough, it also automatically connects callers to the florists.

This ability to interact with other computer applications means that AT&T can customize its 800 service to handle many of the functions now handled internally by a company. These services can automatically fax product information to a number the caller provides, print mailing labels, and even instruct a warehouse to ship the product and print the invoice.

Going Global

While network-based systems can make even a small company a marketing powerhouse, today's increasingly global economy demands that 800 service set its sights beyond the United States. Since AT&T started offering international 800 numbers in 1984, the number of countries where the service is available has grown to 67. It is expected to double in the next few years.

Around the world, 800-like services continue to multiply, although less rapidly than in the United States. In France, Italy, Norway, and Denmark, they're known as "green number" services; in Japan, where toll-free calling was introduced only a few years ago, 800 calls are known as "auto-collect calls"; and in Germany, 800 numbers are called "130 service." In Canada, where toll-free calling accounts for approximately 20 percent of all calls, the trend in toll-free calling appears to be following the same explosive growth as its U.S. counterpart. In France and Germany, the number is less than 10 percent.

Although 800 services still account for only a small percentage of international telephone calls, many businesses, including mail-order companies, airlines, travel agencies, and management consulting firms, are beginning to use the service to gain a foothold in foreign markets without having to open a branch.

For example, Myrtle Beach Golf Holiday, a non-profit cooperative that promotes golf vacations to the world-famous area of South Carolina, has used an international 800 number to attract hundreds of thousands of visitors from around the world, including Sweden, Norway, Denmark, Ireland, Japan, and the Netherlands.

And foreign languages no longer need be a barrier to completing a sale for U.S. businesses. When a non-English-speaking caller phones Myrtle Beach, services such as AT&T's Language Line® kick in. Language Line provides 24-hour-a-day interpretation services for 140 languages.

International 800 service and the full spectrum of today's offerings—and tomorrow's—will enable business people to operate anywhere on earth. Mobility and the ability to fully complete business transactions are expected to launch 800 service into another phase of rapid growth. Callers will routinely shop by using pictures and computer information received on devices that are rapidly moving off the drawing board to general availability.

As businesses continue seeking new ways to reach and service customers, toll-free 800 service will remain one of technology's most remarkable—and flexible—inventions.

–12–
ELECTRONIC MARKETING 2000

Cecil C. Hoge, Sr.

Cecil C. Hoge, Sr., is Chairman of Harrison-Hoge Industries, Inc., and of Hubert Hoge & Sons Advertising, Inc. He is the author of *Mail Order Moonlighting, Mail Order Know-How, What We Can Learn from the Century of Completion Between Sears and Wards: The First 100 Years Are the Toughest,* and *The Electronic Marketing Manual,* as well as countless shorter pieces and works-in-progress. He has been interviewed on over 1,000 radio and television stations, in various publications, and on line, and has lectured extensively, as well.

In *The Electronic Marketing Manual*, I define *electronic marketing* (EM) as "any transfer of goods or services from seller to buyer (the broadest definition of marketing) that involves one or more electronic methods or media.

Electronic Marketing Is Not New

Electronic buying and selling started by telegraph in the 19th century, over 152 years ago. Telephone marketing is now over 100 years old; radio over 72 years; broadcast TV almost half a century; and cable over 25 years. With the advent and mass acceptance of telephone, radio, TV, and cable, electronic media have become the dominant marketing force. New permutations of these four electronic methods as well as the microcomputer explosion continue to create many new forms of electronic media.

The evolution of each dominant marketing medium and method into newer, more effective forms is well known. Telegraphed sales proposals, the first interactive form of electronic marketing, let to proposals by telex, then by fax, and by electronic mall (E-mail). Likewise, commercials on records led to those on film and later on audiotape, and then videotape.

The power of electronic marketing to sell is not new; neither is its dominant role in all marketing and its ability to mesh with and make more effective other forms of marketing. What is new is the accelerated pace of change of electronic media and methods. How does EM affect your business and career now?

The power of older electronic and print media (when used in the same old way) is fading. Shotgun telemarketing irritates more than it sells. Telephone tag wastes time and money. Fragementation of TV audience and viewer fatigue from too many commercials fritters away effectiveness as ad rates rise. Minutes spent reading publication and direct mail shrink, while trust in ad claims drops. Meanwhile, new

---

Futurescope

Communication is now telescoping into perhaps a tenth of the time the scope and variety and universality of change that transportation underwent in the last two centuries. It's coming faster than any previous technological revolution. As the EM marketing-communications revolution nears the year 2000, it is moving into tidal-wave speed and driving out of business marketers who do not join in. How will EM affect you between now and then? It need not hurt you, it can help you greatly, and it can be far easier to adapt to than people unfamiliar with it now fear.

research, targeting, enhancement, technology, media, and ways to integrate it all more effectively make EM more profitble than ever before—for those who know how. But most don't, and fewer still keep up with emerging EM media and methods.

Which of These Electronic Marketing Forms Do You Now Use?

Audiotext
Voice Mail
Talking ads
Sponsored Telemedia
Inbound and outbound faxmail
Fax-aided ads
Video brochures
Video demos
Video catalogs
Commercials in videocassettes
Video premiums

Ads in movies on planes
Interactive catalogs on computer
   disks
Electronic data interchange (EDI)
Electronic mail (E-mail)
Information and entertainment
   computer networks (e.g.,
   CompuServe)
Computer bulletin boards (BBSs)
Online catalogs
Online marketplaces

How Familiar Are You with These Forms?

Electronic marketing machines in
   kiosks at stores and trade shows
Automatic teller machines (ATMs)
Interactive catalogs and market-
   places on CD-ROM
Instore radio and TV
Couponing machines

Computerized signage
TV shopping networks
Direct by satellite (dbs) business
   television
Audio- and teleconferencing
Interactive electronic vending

Which of These Best Suit Your Near-Future Needs?

EM-aided PR
TV infomercials
EM-aided sales force
EM-aided export
EM-aided store

EM-aided telemarketing
EM-aided direct marketing
EM classified ads
EM home office
EM moonlighting

EM change is racing faster! New EM technology is falling in price while increasing sales. The cost per thousand of new EM media shows on the graph in a line constantly curving downward. Another line of constantly inflating costs of present methods keeps curving upward. Soon, on the graph, the two lines will meet—the fatal fade-out kiss for much marketing as we now know it. The next six years can bring to a peak the most sweeping changes to date. What will EM be like?

Predictions of Top Authorities about EM

There are going to be more channels available to the point of infinity. There won't be a limitation on the number of channels. We will reach that point in the next decade.
> —Charles Dolan, founder of Cablevision, Inc., one of the biggest
> multiple system operators (MSOs) in the world

When television becomes digital, customers can pick and choose...by 1999 40 million TV households will be digital.
> —Joe Collins, CEO, Time-Warner

By the turn of the century the average PC will be more powerful than today's supercomputer.

But the end of the decade multimedia PCs could easily account for a third or more of total (PC) sales....Business software will also go multimedia. Documents will have text, drawings, video clips and speech. E-mail will become e-mail/voice mail. Databases will store text, graphics, images, speech and so on.

It is much harder to project the capabilities of PCs for the year 2000, but it is worth a try.... The color display will have a 1,024 × 768 resolution and will be HDTV compatible ... the home PC will have advanced multimedia features including a special processor that will compress and decompress images, recognize handwriting and speech input and generate speech music and sounds....The optical disk will be able to read music CDs. CD-ROMs and erasable optical disks. Handwriting input and speech recogniation will be included.... (Multimedia) Software that's the equivalent of an expert in nearly every field such as lawyer, doctor, accountant, or financial planner will be common.

At the end of the decade virtual reality (VR)... in some ways the next generation of multimedia—could have a major impact on computer applications.

The availability of wireless communication to any computer anywhere in the world will make personal digital assistands (PDAs), sub-notebooks and notebook computers indispensable for many people in a few years ... a steep cost decline will make the technology prevalent by the end of this decade ... a nd the annual shipments may then surpass 100 mill units.
> —Egil Juliussen, cofounder of *Future Computing,* in the 1993
> *Computer Industry Almanac,* which he and his wife Karen founded

Barcode scanning, telephone message unit data, interactive TV will provide marketers with a goldmine of information. We'll see the emergence of new market research firms, geared toward information processing and forecasting instead of information gathering.
—Robert A. Fox, CEO of Continental Can Co.

The curve of growth for computer messaging will go almost straight up. Electronic mail will replace mass postal mailings.
—Alexander Lippit, Jr., Arthur Andersen & Co.

Computerized trading will inevitably replace stock exchanges.
—DuWayne Peterson, top technology executive at Merrill Lynch

Videotext will take off and soon in the new century over half of U.S. homes will have it and using it will be as natural as using a telephone.
—Gary Arlen, founder of *The Interactivity Report*

Others have predicted the following for the years between now and the new century: 2.45 billion people will use computers by the year 2000, or even sooner. Everything from Broadway shows to business seminars might be offered by PPV technology. TV will be programmed like a computer, interactive and completely personalized. High-definition television (HDTV) programs and movies with much sharper TV images and picture quality much closer to that of a movie screen will be distributed via VCR, video disk, optical/electrical cable system, DBS, and terrestrial transmission.

More custom, personalized TV newspapers. Far more global electronic marketing via DBS, satellite radio, shortwave radio, unwired networks, syndicated shows, and network chains. Voice print identification, like fingerprints, to order by phone. Custom smart cards that eliminate processing of tickets and reservations for anything. More ethnic and multilanguage TV and radio: by C-band and Ku-band, DBS and microband, UHF and VHF, and by cable. More kiosk networks for advertisers, first local, then regional, then national.

Most purchase orders will be electronic. Computer auctions will multiply. Many more advertisers will send coupons directly into the home. Far more customers will pay electronically. Electronic transfers will grow to several times the current percentage of check transfers.

Electronic marketing does not eliminate selling, advertising, and marketing; most kinds of media that have been profitably used in the past; or most kinds of businesses and careers that now exist. Rather, EM will create opportunities for entirely new careers and businesses. It does not negate the basic sound strategy of dealing with others for maximum mutual benefit and profit. It simply gives rich rewards to those who sell and advertise and market in new ways (as each is proven successful). Those who use the new ways effectively will outcompete and leave behind those who don't.

Between now and the year 2000, what can you do to ride the EM wave to your greatest benefit and profit and not be blown away by it? Consider what railroads can teach us about electronic opportunity. The first giant fortunes came to those who made railroads happen, but only after surviving the Darwinian struggle of the speculative period when most failed and before ever-growing government regulation. Compare them to media owners. Next came the suppliers to railroads of rails, trains, coal, and even railroad watches and uniforms. Consider them the peripherals. Then came the joint ventures worked out with the suppliers of dining cars, sleeping cars, refrigerator cars, and express companies. Think of them as software. Along with them came suppliers to them and to the railroads, such as the steel industry.

But all this made possible farm belts and much bigger cities, suburbs, and metro areas. Expanded postal service in turn led to a mammoth increase in the numbers of newspapers and their circulation and the meteoric rise of national magazines on a vast scale, which created the first volume advertising locally, regionally, and then nationally; and national sales forces and national distribution of products; and powerful giant wholesalers, department stores, and huge mail order catalogs.

And all this made possible explosive growth in sales and profits for makers of most kinds of products. These manufacturers knew or learned how to take advantage of the new conditions (from tiny start-ups and moonlighters to big companies and those in between). Employees who helped their companies grow in the new ways kept their jobs and got good raises or did better elsewhere or started their own enterprises. Those that did not acquire the new know-how lagged behind and did not survive. In the end, more fortunes macro to mini (and many times the total made by the railroad owners and suppliers) were made by the marketers astute enough to know how to benefit most from the changed conditions, in the way most practical and profitable for each. The same thing happened in each major technological breakthrough, from electricity to the automobile industry.

Changing Electronic Opportunities: Which Are Best for You?

With every sea change in electronic marketing and media, from the telegraph to the telephone to radio and television and movies and computers and PCs, more astute marketers made change work for them, and those who clung to the old methods were at an increasing disadvantage, often one too great to continue to compete successfully, stay in business, or keep their jobs.

Despite its complexity, the marketing communications revolution is easier to adapt to than the marketing transportation revolution, because it is a speeded-up evolution of numerous forms, some of which will affect your business and career faster than others. The primary way to adapt is via EM know-how, which can be acquired gradually.

Study EM Successes and Failures

Learn what works as well as potential pitfalls. Keep a file of EM failures, but also note any successful resurrection later of EM near-successes. Seek out warnings, tips, and advice from smart EM entrepreneurs, consultants, and vendors. Investigate dangers and seek expert opinions about special EM opportunities. Look for EM business jackpots that fit you: new products, services, and businesses only possible because of new changes in present forms of EM and the rise and proliferation of new forms.

However much your present EM know-how, keep adding more. Whatever your EM specialty, also become an EM generalist. However little you know, fear not to start with the EM basics. You'll quickly find your EM assets, what is easier for you to learn and where your past experience, hobbies, and interests give you a special edge. In any case, make a hobby of learning more about EM. Exchange EM information with others. Get the EM learning habit, starting with a little each day.

Section III
Customer Service Strategies

Every business owes its existence to its customers, and developing and implementing strategies that meet their customers' needs and demands is vital to every organization's success.

In "Proactive Servicing for Competitive Advantage," Richard Chvala explores how companies can use technologies that will help answer the seemingly eternal question: "What does the customer really want?" Michael Herrington outlines the various levels of customer satisfaction and how a company can develop new methods to assess and improve customer satisfaction levels in "The Hierarchy of Customer Satisfaction." As the world moves toward a global marketplace U.S. companies would do well to measure their customer service performance on a worldwide scale. So argue Allen Paison and Jeffrey Marr in "Perception Is Still All There Is: Getting the Customer in Focus." Next Sybil Stershic reminds us that while a global perspective is important, so is marketing on the "home front." In "Internal Marketing: Building Customer Satisfaction from the Inside Out," she focuses on an often-overlooked "market"—one's own colleagues—and demonstrates how improved internal marketing can improve overall marketing effectiveness. And in "Service Blueprinting," G. Lynn Shostack outlines the newest way to plan for success by organizing the customer service function to achieve maximum results.

–13–

PROACTIVE SERVICING FOR COMPETITIVE ADVANTAGE

Richard J. Chvala

Richard J. Chvala serves as an adjunct professor at the University of Richmond School of Business Management. He is Senior Consultant, Sales and Marketing Training, for Ethyl Corporation, a Fortune 500 company based in Richmond, Virginia. Chvala also serves on the national board of the American Marketing Association, and was the keynote speaker at the AMA's First International Congress on Customer Satisfaction. Rich has more than 15 years of experience as a national sales manager and marketing executive for both capital goods and service companies. Chvala's training specialties include strategic selling, customer communications, and creating value for the customer. He is the co-author of *Total Quality and Marketing*. Chvala received his undergraduate degree in biochemistry from Michigan Technological University and his M.B.A. from Michigan.

A few companies are attempting a new tactic to differentiate themselves from competitors. This new approach, *proactive servicing,* has been used quite successfully in service markets, and it is directly transferable to industrial markets. Here's how it works: The business marketer must first analyze the firm's position given these simple questions:

1. What does the customer want?

2. What does our firm do best?

3. What is the competition offering?

If 2 matches 1 better than 3 matches 1, then you have a competitive advantage. This analytical process has been available since the dawn of marketing. However, the firms that conduct the best research in each of these areas will indisputably come out on top.

In Figure 1, the inner circle represents the features or benefits of the core product. Expanding outward, you'll find primary services, reactive services, and, finally, proactive services. A good illustration of proactive servicing is in the airline industry.

The core product offered by airlines is a seat, from point A to point B. And, although we all have joked about the airlines' primary level of services, it is, simply, a reservation for transportation and a way to remit payment. Note that assigned seating is not necessarily a primary service. Some airlines offered just a boarding pass, and others, until recent years, accepted only cash for payment. Most primary levels of service might be considered simply what the Federal Aviation Administration requires: a seat, a seatbelt, an oxygen mask, and a flotation device if water is traversed.

Reactive services include those items that develop out of competition. For the airline industry, these services have ranged from boarding passes, advanced yet restricted discount fares, peanuts and other choice refreshments, all the way to the frequent flyer program and preferred status upgrades.

Futurescope

Many successful industrial or business-to-business companies have discovered that market segmentation is fundamental to increasing profitability. However, in today's international arena, that strategy alone cannot withstand the warlike onslaught brought about by global competition. Emerging technologies will allow the sales force and market researchers to get to the heart of the question, "What does the customer want?"

Figure 1   Proactive Services Model

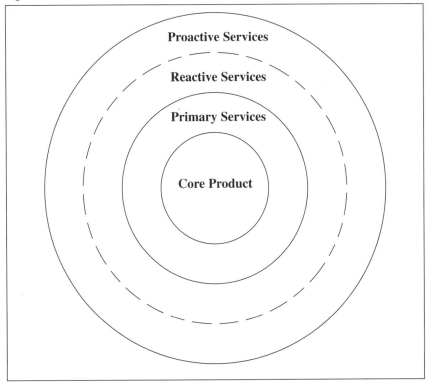

Seasoned business travelers will recall that American Airlines initiated the frequent flyer program in 1981, and it took more than 6 months for the major competitors to follow suit. The service model relationship demonstrates that each reactive service was once a proactive service. When an airline tries something new to lure travelers, the more successful ideas are quickly copied. Virtually all airlines now offer frequent flyer programs. When American launched its AAdvantage program in 1981, it possessed a competitive advantage not shared by other airlines for several months; therefore it was a proactive service.

In today's fast-paced, competitive world, very few competitive moves last long. News travels fast, and customers expect parallel reaction. During the 1992 holiday season, an airline advertised an offer of double frequent flyer mileage for most routes. The very next day, several other airlines matched that program.

Unfortunately, when the competition matches your proactive service it reverts back into the reactive service circle. At that level, it becomes a service that all customers expect, at no additional charge—a potential disadvantage rather than a competitive edge (no additional profit).

One airline recently attempted a significant proactive service. It followed the rules in researching questions 1,2, and 3 of competitive advantage, and it discovered that what the business traveler really valued was first-class seating at coach fares. This airline, Eastern, realized that (a) it was losing business travelers rapidly, due to its financial mess, (b) it had many planes on the ground, providing a high inventory of vacant first-class seats, and (c) that first-class seats for coach prices was something that business travelers cherished.

The offer was "Pay coach, fly first class." That offer went unmatched for several months and gained over 7 percent of the business traveler market share. Although Eastern eventually went bankrupt, insiders give credit to that proactive service for keeping the airline alive longer than industry projections. Perhaps it was too little, too late, but there is another airline offering that unmatched service today.

The key to discovering the best proactive services is to imagine a service that your customer wants and that competition either cannot match in technology or ability or elects not to match due to management constraints, lack of market knowledge, or other reasons. Such an effort is likely to provide a competitive advantage.

Let's examine a real-life, industrial case. Company A and Company B each have elected to sell chemical products in the same market. Both have discovered that customers desire a "guaranteed" inventory for just in time (JIT) production management. Customers in this market fear a plant shutdown if this feedstock inventory is depleted. Company A offers to service the market by providing special storage tanks for its chemical on-site for the customer. The tanks are purchased, installed, and maintained by the supplier—a relatively small investment to assure a strategic partnership.

Company B's market share begins to suffer. Company B has a choice, either to match Company A and also offer storage tanks, or to further research the market to discover true needs. If Company B matches the offer of Company A, then there is no competitive advantage, and the proactive service (the storage tanks) falls back into the reactive service circle and becomes an expected service by all customers.

However, Company B, rather than offering to install tanks in a "me-too" move, elects to offer a computer-assisted inventory monitor, which, by the customer's examination, is actually a better, more efficient system of inventory control without the burden of extra storage tanks on the customer's plant site. Eventually, most customers want the service offered by Company B, and Company A soon finds itself with a backlog of special storage tanks and, more importantly, no competitive advantage.

Company B wins, because it stayed proactive rather than reactive. History demonstrated that Company B won in two important categories: return on service investment and increased market share.

The proactive services target model exercise is an easy technique to build a competitive strategy to "out-service" your competition. Just like television, though, do not attempt this strategy unless you are a professional. Remember that the question, "What does your customer want?" is often best answered through a combination of your sales force, an independent market researcher, and the customer's direct input.

—14—
THE HIERARCHY OF CUSTOMER SATISFACTION

Michael Herrington

Michael Herrington, a consultant in total quality management and business process redesign, is based in Fairfield, Connecticut. He has worked with numerous clients in the development and implementation of their quality improvement strategies. Using both the Malcolm Baldridge National Quality Award criteria and the criteria for the Connecticut Award for Excellence, he has led organizational assessments and subsequent implementation of organization quality improvement initiatives. Prior to entering consulting, Herrington was Vice President for Quality Improvement for Olin Corporation. He is a graduate of The Ohio State University, and holds a degree in mechanical engineering.

You've heard the discussions and arguments: "I don't think we should start a quality process until we know what the customer wants." "The customer wants the lowest price and nothing else." "My customer wants partnerships." "I think on-time delivery is more important." "You might think on-time delivery is important, but my customer says he wants more reliable products." If we cannot achieve more understanding of customer needs and satisfaction levels, we will never be able to make the tough decisions required to bring about change and improvement. Because, as we know, a quality initiative that is not inextricably tied to customer satisfaction is doomed to failure. The final arbiter of success is the customer, the final reward for success is profit.

Many business people oversimplify the concept of customer satisfaction. There is a tendency to think in terms of an "average" customer—a customer who wants only one or a few things. This is illogical from two perspectives. First, every business has numerous customers, each of whom at a given time has a unique level of individual satisfaction. Second, each of these unique customers' satisfaction levels is changing over time. So, customer satisfaction is a complex moving target, and a process for determining customer satisfaction has to detect both this complexity and rate of change.

Fortunately, customer satisfaction follows a logical pattern. To understand this pattern, we can use a corollary model of the stages of human satisfaction. Almost 40 years ago, Abraham H. Maslow developed an insightful model of human need, satisfaction, and motivation. Maslow postulated a hierarchy of needs, the satisfaction of which was a primary driver of human behavior. The five basic needs he defined are as follows:

- Physiological

- Safety

- Belongingness

- Esteem

- Self-actualization

Futurescope

Customer satisfaction will be a key component of success in the 21st century, when potential customers will be able to select suppliers from all over the globe, using advanced telecommunications and electronic mail to communicate their needs, complaints, and desires. The forward-looking marketer will learn how to assess and improve customer satisfaction in order to compete in a marketplace without borders.

Maslow believed that these human needs had to be satisfied in a fixed sequence, from physiological to self-actualization. Furthermore, these needs had to be satisfied cumulatively. Thus, if an individual's current motivation is satisfaction of a higher need, such as the need for esteem, the lower needs of physiological, safety, and belongingness must have been, and are currently being, met. But if a lower need, such as safety, is suddenly no longer satisfied, behavior will change. Achieving esteem is no longer a motivator. The individual's behavior and motivation will revert to satisfying the now-unmet need of being safe. Once the individual feels safe again, his or her motivation will then go toward satisfying the next higher need of belongingness. Following satisfaction of the belongingness need, the operative need will again become achievement of esteem.

There is much in Maslow's model that predicts the success or failure of contemporary culture change initiatives. For example, employees worried about job security (safety) might be unresponsive to non-monetary recognition programs (esteem). Employee empowerment initiatives (self-actualization) might not be successful in a culture of low respect for individuals (esteem). Seeking empowerment (self-actualization) without first creating involvement (belongingness) is probably fruitless. Failure to provide assurance of job security (safety) will undermine a quality program that is expected to lead to employee-initiated productivity and organizational streamlining.

Like individuals, customers have an analogous hierarchy of needs. Critical to a successful quality initiative is understanding the customer satisfaction hierarchy and knowing the customer's current need and satisfaction level. This then becomes a framework for assessment and action.

The Stages of Customer Needs

The lowest-level human need is physiological: food, sleep, etc. The analogous customer need is for core products or services to work. If the machine doesn't run, the chemical doesn't react, the flight is cancelled, or the bank doesn't honor our checks, then no other level of customer-supplier relationship matters. This is the most basic need. Your core offering, whether a product or service, must work.

The next higher human need is safety: security, protection, reliability, freedom from anxiety, etc. The customer analog is the need for the set of basic services associated with the core offering (e.g., delivering products on time and undamaged). In a service business, the safety equivalent is accessibility, timely hours of operation, or localized service access. In both product and service businesses, there is need for accurate and reliable invoicing or billing. In price-sensitive businesses, such as industrial products, confidence that the supplier's price is competitive is a safety need. Warranties and guarantees address safety needs by providing a "safety net," backing up a commitment to reliability.

Maslow's third human need, belongingness, equates to a customer's need for an open, accessible, interpersonal, human, two-way relationship. Here we move beyond product and services to the human dimension. Suppliers' employees have to listen to, and communicate with, the customers' employees to understand unique expectations or to solve problems. Examples of customers' "belongingness" needs are frequent sales contact, 800-number assistance services, technical services and customer services to assist in determining which existing product or service offering is right for the customer, and after-sales services.

The fourth need in Maslow's hierarchy is esteem: the human need for acknowledgement, or for having a favorable reputation, prestige, or expertise. In business, suppliers grant the customer prestige and stature by unilaterally committing resources to understanding and anticipating the change forces affecting the customer and then developing new products and/or services. The supplier takes the initiative, and the risk, to present ideas and solutions that the customers themselves might not have realized were possible or valuable.

Maslow's highest need level is self-actualization. The self-actualized individual has the inner knowledge of excellence and mastery in what he or she does. The self-actualized customer relationship has achieved a state of excellence that is often described as a true partnership. The customer has made the supplier a complete and open participant in the detailed, long-term conduct of his or her business. Mastery of the customer's business drives the relationship.

So the customer satisfaction need hierarchy equivalent to Maslow's need hierarchy is as follows:

- Core products and services that work (physiological)

- Basic, reliable services associated with the core products and services (safety)

- Human interaction facilitating selection and use of existing products and services (belongingness)

- Supplier-developed new business solutions (esteem)

- Partnerships (self-actualization)

The Customer Satisfaction Hierarchy at Work

Evidence of the hierarchy of customer needs is seen repeatedly in customer surveys in which customers are asked to declare their most important needs. For example, Eastman Chemical Company's customer surveys established the following ranking of needs:

1. Product quality
2. Product uniformity
3. Supplier integrity
4. Correct delivery
5. Pricing
6. Listening
7. Supplier flexibility
8. Follow-up
9. Pricing response time
10. Product safety
11. Freight practices
12. Credit practices
13. Complaints/Credit
14. Personal relationships
15. Product knowledge
16. Training
17. Order entry
18. Technical service
19. Product stewardship
20. Supplier information

The highest priority need is for basic product quality. Then comes the equivalent of the safety need in correct delivery and pricing. Next are such factors as listening, flexibility, follow-up, and response time, which equate to belongingness needs. Down the list we find items such as training and product stewardship, which equate to esteem, in that the supplier is expected to take initiatives that are in the customer's interest.

Milliken, in its customer surveys, identified the customer hierarchy as follows:

1. Product quality
2. On-time delivery
3. Handling late deliveries
4. Attitude
5. Order lead time
6. Price

Again, we find the evolution from the very basic "things that work" need to higher level needs, such as attitude.

What makes Maslow's needs hierarchy so powerful is its sequential and cumulative nature. So, too, is the hierarchy of customer satisfaction. Thus, the basic need for "things that work" must first be satisfied. Having achieved this, the customer priority and focus then changes to the associated basic services that give greater reliability. Both of these needs having been satisfied, the priority next goes to the interpersonal relationship between the customer and supplier. In this sequence, a supplier will "grow" the relationship with the customer. For example, if a customer has confidence in product quality and uniformity and believes that you will deliver on time and at a competitive price, then:

1. For that customer,

2. At that point in time,

the need for listening becomes increasingly significant. In fact, under these conditions, listening is the most important issue because it is the customer's next most important unsatisfied need. This must become the focus of efforts, because, all lower needs having been satisfied, this is now the number-one unfulfilled customer need.

Because of the cumulative nature of the need hierarchy, if a formerly satisfied lower-level need suddenly becomes unmet, the relationship collapses to the level of the lowest unmet need. If, for example, we are working with a customer at the partnership level and suddenly an existing product or service fails to work, the customer's next immediate need is to be reassured that the supplier's existing basic products and services work. Similarly, if we are trying to introduce a new product or service innovation to a customer, and billing or delivery performance or established products falter, the customer's immediate attention is diverted to solving the billing or delivery problem. In the example above, what happens if, while working to satisfy the customer's need for listening, the company falters in meeting a lower-level, previously satisfied need, such as product delivery? The customer will diminish, if not abandon, the concern for listening, and direct his or her attention back to the now-unsatisfied need for reliable delivery.

Let's complicate matters! Let's introduce competition. What is now important is not the level of customer satisfaction with one supplier, but rather with their best, or normal, suppliers. If a Milliken customer is satisfied with the product quality, delivery performance, and handling of late deliveries from normal suppliers, then this customer's most urgent current need is for supplier employees with positive attitudes. But where are we? Well, if we are still trying to make the sale based on a promise of on-time delivery, we are definitely on the outside looking in. Even worse, if we fell by the wayside at some point in the past by not being competitive in our delivery performance, we are not only outside, we are outside and in a deep hole. Like bringing food to a person who is not hungry, we are advocating a motivator to a customer who no longer has this need. Unless one of the current suppliers falters, we might never get a chance to prove ourselves. Such is the power of market leadership. Having proven that they can do the basics, market leaders alone have the freedom to differentiate themselves through more esoteric offerings.

Implications for Customer Satisfaction Determination and Measurement

How can we make use of the model of the hierarchy of customer satisfaction? On one level it can serve as a touchstone for sales representatives. Since each customer has a specific priority of needs and a particular satisfaction level at any given time, the key sales questions are the following:

- What is the customer's currently operative need level?

- How does the customer rate our performance relative to this, and all lower, need levels?

- How are competitors satisfying the needs to the current operative level?

Establishing and continuously reconfirming this characterization of both the customer and the competitive situation is fundamental to successful selling. Performing this appraisal for each customer allows customers to be unique and individual. Repeating this appraisal frequently leads to understanding the cycle time of changing customer need and satisfaction levels. This establishes the foundation for the kind of "mass customization" that increasingly characterizes markets and market leaders. With the increasing emphasis on flexibility and cycle time reduction, monthly, or at least quarterly, reappraisal is in order.

What are the implications of the hierarchy of customer satisfaction for determination of customer needs and overall customer satisfaction measurement? Fortunately, with regard to the lower-level needs, we don't need a lot of sophisticated market research. It is pretty clear what these needs are: products and services that work, are conveniently available, are delivered on time and undamaged, and are billed correctly. All companies have a great deal of data from the customer on performance against these needs. This data exists in product returns, warranty claims, sales adjustments, and customer complaints. Elementary as this sounds, these sources of measurement of fulfilling lower-level customer needs are much underutilized by senior executives in the United States. A recent study by Ernst & Young found that only 30 percent of U.S. companies rank customer complaints as a major quality measure. In contrast, 60 percent of Japanese and German companies heavily utilize customer complaint measurement. Recognizing that satisfaction of lower-level customer needs is a precondition to differentiation based on the more esoteric higher-level needs, this is an amazing statistic. If a company doesn't have the basics down, it is wasting its time in trumpeting its fringe benefits. This is equivalent to offering praise to an individual who is concerned about where his next meal is coming from.

At the intermediate need levels—the interpersonal relationship with customers and taking new initiatives to solve customer problems—the determination of satisfaction is more difficult. Here we are dealing with more subjective matters. The line between determining satisfaction and determining new or unfulfilled expectation becomes fuzzy. In industrial businesses, there are multiple sources of information from the customer. The customer's employee who can tell us if our products work is probably a different individual than the one who can tell us about the attitude and helpfulness of our employees. Unavoidably, we now have to use techniques such as surveys, customer focus groups, and analyses of gain and loss of customers.

Determining the final stage of customer satisfaction—partnership—is straightforward. Either you are partners or you are not. If you are, chances are you are nearly sole-sourced, have the earliest knowledge of evolving customer business plans, and are on the inside track for participating in the customer's growth and prosperity. You have satisfied, and continue to satisfy, all the needs on the customer's hierarchy of need and satisfaction. As long as you continue to do so, your competitive advantage, and your future, should be secure.

So what does the customer want? In the long run, everything! But what the customer wants now is dependent on what satisfaction level is currently being met. By meeting these customer needs sequentially and cumulatively, we ultimately will give the customer everything and will become the partner on the inside rather than the suitor on the outside.

–15–
PERCEPTION IS
STILL ALL THERE IS
Getting the Customer
in Focus

Allen R. Paison and Jeffrey W. Marr

Allen R. Paison is President and CEO of Walker: Customer Satisfaction Measurements. Prior to joining Walker in 1983, he worked for NFO Research and Xerox Corporation. Mr. Paison speaks regularly on the topic of customer satisfaction measurement in domestic and international marketing. He is on the Boards of Advisors of the First Interstate Center for Service Marketing (Arizona State University), the Institute for the Study of Business Markets (Penn State University), and the Center for Customer-Driven Quality (Purdue University), and is Trustee of the Marketing Sciences Institute.

Jeffrey W. Marr joined Indianapolis-based Walker Research in 1977 and is now Vice President, Client Services. He has ultimate responsibility for a variety of W:CSM (Walker Customer Service Management) national and multinational accounts. He holds a B.A. from Indiana University. He is a member of the American Marketing Association, the American Society for Quality Control, the Conference Board and the Marketing Science Institute.

The Growth of Customer Satisfaction Measurement into the 21st Century

Back in 1986, we noted that the number of companies formally measuring customer satisfaction was entirely too small. After all, many had already lost market share dramatically. However, as many CEOs confessed to Tom Peters at that time, business leaders were not putting their customer measures "where their mouth was."[1] Most were still managing on financial measures and internal quality assessment much more than using the perceptions of their customers for direction.

We are pleased to now recognize the progress that businesses in America and elsewhere have made in deploying customer satisfaction measurement programs. Evidence of this progress is most clearly demonstrated in research findings from the 1992 Ernst & Young/American Quality Foundation *International Quality Study*. Within the context of the study, when business people from Canada, Germany, Japan, and the United States are asked the importance of customer satisfaction, there is a dramatic growth in customer satisfaction as a primary criterion in the strategic planning process in companies in all countries.[2] The growth percentages are substantial, therefore reinforcing the commitment to a formal customer satisfaction measurement process (see Figure 1).

A second set of information from the *International Quality Study* observes growth in the use of quality as an assessment criterion for senior management compensation. Again, we find substantial growth across all countries on the use of quality as a compensation variable for senior management (see Figure 2). Given the relationship between quality and customer satisfaction (perception is all there is), one would have to forecast a solid future for professionally managed customer satisfaction measurement processes in the years to come.

But Why Aren't All Companies Formally Measuring Customer Input? What Is the Major Hurdle?

One key obstacle still appears to be a lack of trust in quality-related data that come from the customer. Some might argue that customer perceptions do not necessar-

Futurescope

As marketers look forward to the new century, they would do well to examine international business practices. As U.S. companies increasingly compete head to head with companies based abroad, their customer satisfaction performance will have to measure up to worldwide standards. Comprehensive assessment of customer satisfaction is the first step toward success in the global marketplace.

Figure 1   Percentage of Businesses Indicating the Importance of
Customer Satisfaction as a Primary Criterion in the
Strategic Planning Process

	Past (last 3 years)	Current	Future (Next 3 Years)
Canada	20%	44%	80%
Germany	10%	22%	59%
Japan	30%	42%	80%
United States	18%	37%	69%

Source: Ernst & Young (America Quality Foundation *International Quality Study*).

ily reflect the "real" quality of products and services. But, to paraphrase Peters and Austin and others, what else really counts besides perception, if that's the stuff on which purchase decisions are based?

As Peters says, "Perception is all there is." What customers perceive is real; it must be listened to and acted on.

Translating into Hard Data

But let us go a step further with this business about perceptions. Many managers perceive that customer feedback tends to be "soft data" for which they would cringe at being held accountable. This perception is another reality that must be dealt with. This does not mean avoiding customer input; that input is crucial. Rather, there is a need to translate soft customer input into a hard-nosed, quantitative measurement tool that will be credible to management. Customer input

Figure 2   Percentage of Businesses Indicating Primary Importance of Quality as an Assessment Criterion for Senior Management Compensation

	Past (last 3 years)	Current	Future (Next 3 Years)
Canada	8%	15%	35%
Germany	2%	18%	39%
Japan	19%	28%	31%
United States	10%	19%	51%

Source: Ernst & Young (America Quality Foundation *International Quality Study*).

should be obtained from a survey program that is viewed as an objective, consistent, and reliable tool for managers.

Once the carefully designed external program is put in place, even the most hard-bitten members-oriented managers become believers in the importance and potential of customer feedback.

Many of the methods used in internal quality assurance, such as probability sampling and ongoing data collection, have been successfully employed to develop dynamic, external quality monitoring programs for companies large and small. The following basic principles for designing a quantitative customer satisfaction measurement process have not really changed since the 1980s.

1. **The program should have a dual purpose of providing both a performance measurement and a diagnostic tool.** In other words, the program will be most meaningful if it not only tracks indices of customer satisfaction, but also points out your company's strengths and weaknesses. Practical yet quantitative question scales provide meaningful performance-rating results, while

open-ended probing-type questions help explain the attitudes. In short, the program must be measurable as well as actionable.

2. **The basis for the program is probability sampling of current customers.** The customer population could consist of either the end users of the product (goods or service) or intermediaries in the distribution channel, or both. Once the population is identified, random probability samples are taken to identify the people to be interviewed. Sample size can be planned based on the desired precision and confidence level of the results.

3. **Sampling a mix of long-term customers and new buyers usually proves most useful.** This allows the data to be grouped separately.

   • Those customers who received their first impression of your company's quality during the selling, installation, and set-up activities.

   • Long-term customers who tend to have a different perspective on quality than do new customers.

4. **The program should be designed to be continuous.** Monthly surveys are ideal; quarterly or semiannually are the minimum recommended. As with internal quality control, the continuous program helps keep one's finger on the pulse of performance, measures any seasonal changes, and can provide an early warning system of quality changes. Providing frequent reports of customer opinion also emphasizes the importance of the program in the minds of employee and staff.

5. **Telephone surveys usually provide the best all-around method of collecting data from customers.** Unfortunately, in survey research, a random probability sample selection does not also guarantee that the results are representative of the population. Those who respond might or might not have similar characteristics as those who choose not to respond. In these circumstances, telephone contact produces a more random data set than does a mail-out, self-administered questionnaire, at least relative to customer satisfaction issues. This is largely because those who take the time to respond to a mail survey often feel strongly about the issues at hand, so you get very polarized responses. Those who are more neutral on the subject might not fill out a questionnaire, but will often participate in a telephone survey. Personal interviews provide another option, but they have their own logistics—and cost—problems.

6. **It is important to track customers' repurchase intent and willingness to recommend your company to another person, as well as the customer's perception of quality.** From a marketing standpoint, a satisfied customer is more likely to speak well of your company and purchase from you again than

is a dissatisfied customer. Tracking such areas can help your company estimate relative cost of quality for performance in specific aspects of customer perception.

7. **Include in the customer survey the entire array of product and service attributes that determine customer satisfaction and purchase behavior.** Only by taking a comprehensive approach in the survey can your company make a useful diagnosis of strengths and weaknesses. Determining what to include usually requires some exploratory research, such as in-depth individual or group interviews with a small number of customers. Ultimately, external measurements can be linked with internal measurements.

8. **Perform a statistical analysis that evaluates the relative impact of customer requirements as well as your performance in these areas.** Determine the impact of different customer requirements on satisfaction resource-planning decisions. These results can be shown in a quality priority quadrant (see Figure 3), which positions each attribute based on its combined performance and satisfaction impact values.

   It is important to use statistical measures that go beyond just asking customers what they think is important. The things that customers say are important are not always the things that determine what the customers buy. For

Figure 3   Quality Priorities

Critical Improvement High Impact/Low Score	**Leverageable Opportunities** High Impact/Low Score
Low Impact/Low Score **Lesser Weaknesses**	Low Impact/High Score **Lesser Strengths**

example, the recent book *Services Marketing* reports that airline passengers ranked safety as most important. But since most major U.S. airlines are safe, safety did not influence consumer choice among major carriers. Instead, the attributes of lesser important in customer opinion were of highest importance in the marketplace. These aspects are called determinant attributes—those that determine choice or at least word-of-mouth advertising.[3] There are various multivariate techniques for establishing the relative importance of determinant attributes.[4] These have also been termed *driver models,* as they rank-order attributes that "drive" customer satisfaction and behavior.

9. **Competitive quality and customer-satisfaction benchmarks should be used to establish your company's relative quality position in the market.** Once a quantitative study is up and running, the instrument can be modified slightly to gather data from customers of competitors. This data becomes the benchmark that determines whether there are any competitive gaps in the marketplace, attribute by attribute. Of course, a gap in any highly important attribute calls for immediate action.

10. **Provide an avenue for identifying any customer-specific problems.** During the course of interviews with large numbers of customers, it is natural that a few will relate existing problems that have not been reported previously. A follow-up procedure should be established in conjunction with the survey in order to service these customers properly.

11. **Put the survey results to work every day.** Collecting and analyzing data won't have much impact unless findings are regularly discussed and acted on. Up front, with the design of a customer satisfaction program, the following structure should be put into place.

    • Quality review sessions or teams should be identified at three different levels throughout the company. An executive group uses the results to allocate resources and provide direction. Middle management groups focus on customer priorities in the data and help equip the line functions. The line people (who may already belong to quality circles or be involved in other participative management approaches) examine the findings and communicate back up the line what can be done to improve performance.

    • The data from a consistently administered customer quality program can be tied directly to staff and employee incentive plans. Because of their responsibility for allocation of resources, executives should have their salaries and bonuses weighted more heavily by the customer input than line employees.

    • The internal quality assurance administrators should regularly receive customer input so that internal quality systems can be developed to promote the quality aspects that are most important to customers.

External customer satisfaction measurement programs are not intended to replace internal measurements of quality. Rather, they should serve to augment the total quality assurance effort. The internal measures are usually the fastest and best ways to know whether things are being done right. However, to know whether you are doing the *right things* right, you must let the customer be the judge.

Notes

1. Tom Peters and Nancy Austin, *A Passion for Excellence* (New York: Random House, 1985), p. 87.

2. Ernst & Young (America Quality Foundation *International Quality Study*).

3. Christopher H. Lovelock, *Services Marketing* (Englewood Cliffs, N.J.: Prentice Hall, 1984), p. 137.

4. Fred N. Kerlinger and Elazar J. Pedhazur, *Multiple Regression in Behavior Research* (New York: Holt, Rinehart and Winston, 1973). p. 64.

–16–

INTERNAL MARKETING

Building Customer Satisfaction from the Inside Out

Sybil F. Stershic

Sybil F. Stershic is President of Quality Service Marketing, a marketing consulting firm specializing in service quality management training and marketing planning for service and nonprofit organizations. Stershic has extensive experience in services marketing, having held key management positions in advertising, marketing communications, and sales at several commercial banks ranging from $500 million to more than $2 billion in assets. She also served as an instructor of both marketing and management communications at Lehigh University, and is serving her third term on the international board of directors of the American Marketing Association, where she is currently Vice President of Marketing Management.

By its nature, marketing is externally focused. Most of its activities are directed at reaching markets and customers. However, no organization will be successful without the support of its most valuable internal resource: its employees. Hence the need for internal marketing, defined here simply as meeting the needs of employees so they can meet the needs of their customers.

Research has shown customer attitudes, intentions, and perceptions are affected by what employees experience in their organizations. In managing what has been called the employee-customer "mirror"—"the way your employees feel is the way your customers will feel"—internal marketing is applied to ensure a corporate culture that instills customer-focused values in all employees.

Internal Marketing as
a Management Strategy

Despite its name, internal marketing is more a management strategy than a marketing function. According to Christian Grönroos of the Swedish School of Economics, one of internal marketing's early advocates, internal marketing has two basic management components:

- **Attitude Management:** The process of motivating employees to buy in to corporate goals.

- **Communications Management:** Managing the information that employees need to perform effectively.

In this context, internal marketing can be viewed as an umbrella concept for a range of internal activities used in the management of attitudes and communications, including (but not limited to) training, recognition, empowerment, man-

---

Futurescope

Continuing advancements in information technology in the 21st century will allow us to develop and deliver customized products and services to targeted markets. Despite the increasing role of technology in marketing, firms will still depend heavily on employees to interact with customers—whether directly in customer contact positions or behind the scenes in supportive roles. Internal marketing is the management strategy that will be applied to instill customer focus and achieve the necessary balance between "high tech" and "high touch."

agement support, sharing of information, and team building. Elements of both attitude and communications management are found in the following examples of key internal marketing strategies, which focus on the corporate mission, the employee-customer link, international communications, and leadership.

Maximizing the Corporate Mission

As a concise statement that embodies a firm's culture, a corporate mission or vision statement is the single best source to communicate to employees what the organization is all about and what it is striving to achieve. Internal marketing leverages the mission in two ways: first, by making the mission *real* and second, by taking advantage of all opportunities to reinforce the mission.

Typically, firms develop and introduce customer-focused missions with great fanfare. They feature the new mission in employee publications, display framed copies throughout offices, and even distribute plaques or wallet-size versions to all employees. But developing and disseminating the mission are not enough to generate employee buy-in.

Most missions couldn't pass the "That's nice, but what does it really mean?" test. A mission statement is not meaningful unless it is made real and applicable from the employee's perspective. This involves translating the mission into specific, measurable behaviors. Consider the following exercise:

Our mission statement is [fill in your company's actual mission] , which means [fill in the appropriate behaviors based on customer expectations and internal standards] .

For example, a teller who is hired at the Friendliest National Bank is told to provide the friendliest service in town, a rather vague charge. However, at the bank's orientation program, the teller is given the following explanation:

Our tellers are expected to provide the friendliest service in town, *which means* that when a customer approaches your window, you make eye contact with that customer, greet him or her appropriately, use the customer's name during the transaction, offer to discuss any new services the customer might need, thank the customer, and use an appropriate close.

Only when employees clearly understand what is expected of them in fulfilling the mission—when the mission is made real and meaningful—can they start to internalize it. Assuming training is provided (as needed) that enables employees to perform accordingly and the appropriate behaviors are included in performance evaluation, internal marketing can then be applied in its second phase to reinforce the mission.

Once the mission is made real, the next step is to use every opportunity to explain it, repeat it, and demonstrate it in communications with employees. Most companies have a variety of internal media available, such as memos, employee newsletters, staff meetings, orientation and training programs, and bulletin boards, which can be used to share information on how to live up to the mission and to recognize employees who are successful in providing customer satisfaction.

Communicating and reinforcing the mission can start even before new employees are hired. To generate initial awareness, one firm posts its mission where potential new hires can see it when completing job application forms. Upon hiring, new employees receive a letter from the company president welcoming them and their contribution to fulfilling the mission.

Orientation and training programs are also utilized to introduce and explain the corporate mission to new employees. Again, these have little impact if the mission is not made meaningful from the employee's perspective. Internal marketing can be used to take the mission beyond a mere statement and maximize its effectiveness as a dynamic guide for how the company operates and what employees are expected to do.

Ensuring the Employee-Customer Link

To instill customer-focused values in an organization, ALL employees must be linked to the customer, not just those with customer contact or customer service in their job descriptions. Knowing what is expected of them in fulfilling the mission is one way to link employees to customers, but alone it is not enough. In a survey on customer commitment, only 38 percent of the companies that responded said everyone in their organization was aware of what customers do with their company's products or services.

Customer awareness is only part of the problem. Do employees really know and understand who the customer is? To assess this situation, distribute a customer survey to employees and have them complete it as they think the customers would. Comparing their responses to actual customer survey results will indicate how in sync employees really are with customers.

For most organizations, the challenge is finding ways to connect employees who have indirect or no contact with customers. Following are some examples of such efforts:

- Each month, the president of a major food-service company takes a group of employees from its headquarters staff out to lunch at nearby client locations: in the cafeteria or dining facility of a hospital, university, or retirement home.

- The kitchen staff who prepare meals in a nursing home participate in an "Adopt a Resident" program so that they are more personally connected to the results of their efforts.

- A manufacturing firm sends representatives from its maintenance staff out of town to visit clients.

Although companies use different methods to build these linkages, the benefits are the same: employees develop a better awareness and understanding of customers, they feel more valued as part of the corporate team (including new insight and empathy for other employees who have customer contact), and, as a result of being connected to the customer in a tangible way, they strengthen their commitment to serving customers.

Inherent in being customer-focused is the recognition of internal customers: employees serving the needs of other employees who serve the (external) customer. This concept is an integral part of a firm's internal service culture. All employees need to understand who their customers are, whether they are actual consumers or other employees. Studies show that internal service drives external service performance. In organizations where employees take care of each other's business needs, they are more likely to do even better with external customers.

Companies interested in evaluating their internal service culture can conduct in-depth employee research. At a minimum, however, a key question that should be asked to provide critical insight is, "Would you refer a friend to work here?" Results of this employee research will guide an organization in determining how much internal marketing effort is needed to link employees to customers and strengthen the internal service culture.

Minimizing Barriers to Effective Internal Communications

Communication is the foundation of all internal marketing. To be effective, it needs to travel in all directions: top-down, from senior management to all employees; bottom-up, from all levels of employees back up to senior management; and laterally, across all levels of the organization. On the positive side, when employees feel they are in on things they are more likely to become team players. On the other hand, organizational studies found a lack of openness in communications actually reduced employee commitment to organizational goals.

Customer profiles and the results of customer-satisfaction research can be shared using top-down and lateral channels to enable employees to better understand who their customers are and how they feel about the company. In the bottom-up channel, employees can be asked to share any feedback they get from customers as well as provide input on how to improve products and services. Despite the importance of bottom-up and lateral communications for employee involvement, these channels are not being used effectively in organizations.

One study found that 70 percent of employees are afraid to offer their suggestions or ask for clarification for fear of being rejected or chastised. The principle of "no pain, no gain" does little to motivate employees to contribute their ideas to the company. Another study found overall employee dissatisfaction with lateral communications, both between departments as well as within departments.

Clearly, despite a customer-focused mission and the best intentions to create an employee team, organizations cannot be successful until they identify and remove the barriers to their internal communications.

Walking the Talk: Leading by Example

In both word and deed, managers have the opportunity to communicate and reinforce the company's commitment to customers. If executives actually "walk the talk," they send a powerful message to everyone in the organization. Because employees pay close attention to the cues provided by their managers, employees are quick to ascertain the difference between management lip service and commitment, and they respond accordingly. For example, managers who shy away from customer problems cannot expect their employees to go the extra mile in taking care of customers.

Executives who are truly customer-focused also know the value of being accessible to their employees:

- The president of a credit union works as a teller one day a month to spend more time with customers and front-line employees.

- Once a year, the executive staff of a major hotel chain schedules time to work "in the trenches" at its various hotels. The vice president of human resources might work in housekeeping, the president might spend the day as a bellman, and the head of finance might work in the hotel kitchen.

- At a large regional bank, employees are invited to "chat with the chairman" on a designated employee hotline. Both the chairman and president also spend time taking groups of employees to lunch to discuss staff concerns and ideas.

Participating in such activities has numerous benefits. In building empathy with employees, executives are reminded of what it's like to be on the front line. And in receiving management's attention, employees feel more valued. Any effort that brings top management closer to employees also results in strengthening the concept of teamwork and reinforcing common goals.

Not surprisingly, organizations that apply internal marketing note significant improvement in both employee and customer satisfaction. Maximizing the mission, ensuring the employee-customer link, minimizing barriers to effective internal communication, and leading by example are key applications of internal marketing. Using these strategies, as well as any proactive effort to positively impact attitude and communications management, organizations will be able to build customer satisfaction from the inside out.

—17—
SERVICE
BLUEPRINTING

G. Lynn Shostack

G. Lynn Shostack is Chairman, President, and majority owner of Joyce International, Inc., a $200 million company engaged in office products distribution and manufacturing. She is a recognized authority on services marketing, and her award-winning articles have been published in the *Harvard Business Review* and *Journal of Marketing,* as well as in a number of top-selling books. In 1994, Shostack was the first recipient of the Career Contributions Award of the American Marketing Association. She is a summa cum laude graduate of the University of Cincinnati and holds an M.B.A. from Harvard Business School.

Service blueprinting is a method for diagramming an entire service system, so that the entire system can be analyzed, monitored, and understood in terms of effectiveness, efficiency, and quality.

Service blueprinting combines techniques used in industrial engineering, decision theory statistics, consumer and market research, sociology and operations management, none of which alone is adequate for dealing with service system issues.

A basic service blueprint identifies:

1. All the tasks and activities necessary to the performance of the service.

2. The means by which these tasks and activities are rendered.

3. The "evidence" of the service that is presented to the customer and the "enounter points" through which the customer experiences the service (the "Line of Visibility").

4. The facilitating goods and services that support the service system.

When the blueprint has been created, it can then be used for many purposes. A first step would be the costing and quantification of all process steps, a typical "industrial" engineering (now TQM) analysis of time and productivity, which can then be used to improve flows and quality. A second step would be the identification on the blueprint of "fall points" or parts of the process that are critical to customer satisfaction, yet have high "breakdown" rates or potential. These points can then receive corrective design and planning attention to create "fail safe" procedures.

Another use for blueprints is in customer service and market research. The identification of "evidence" and encounter points brings a global view to research and management of consumer interactions with the system as well as coordination of all input to the consumer.

Figures 1–4 illustrate how a basic blueprint may be broken into more and more detailed blueprints until the entire service system has been fully documented.

Futurescope

Every facet of customer service—from defining the tasks necessary for providing first-rate service to measuring internal operations and the levels of customer satisfaction to identifying the internal resources needed to provide exceptional service—is paramount to excellence. Service blueprinting provides a method for improving these operations, both internally and externally.

Figure 1   Summary Blueprint-Office Products Dealer

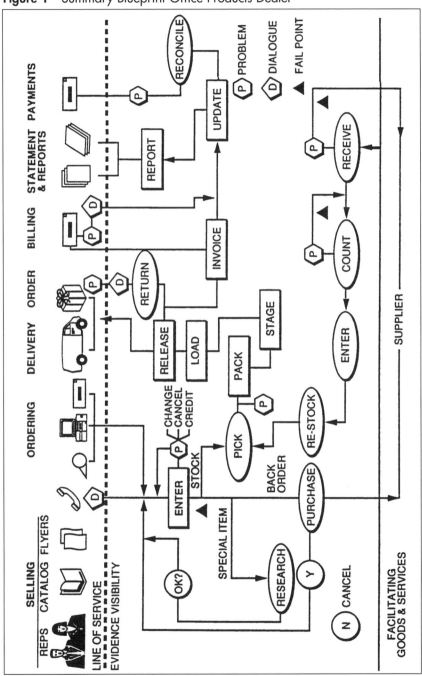

Figure 2   Subsidiary Blueprint-Customer Return

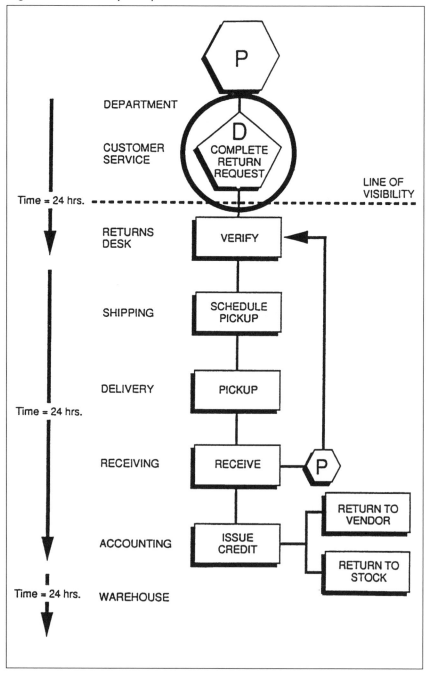

Figure 3   Detailed Blueprint of Dialogue

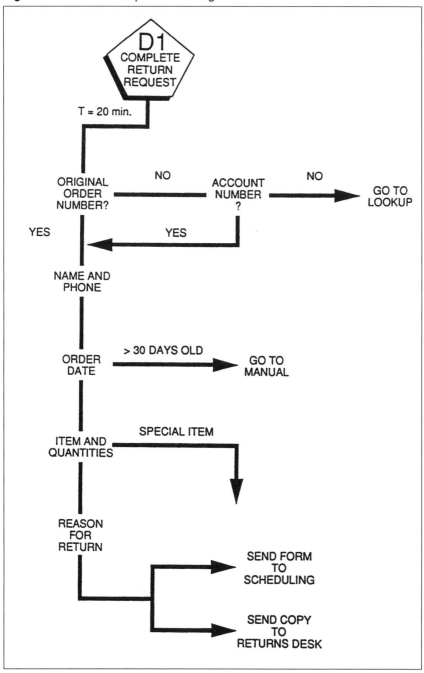

Figure 4   Dialogue Script and Returns Form

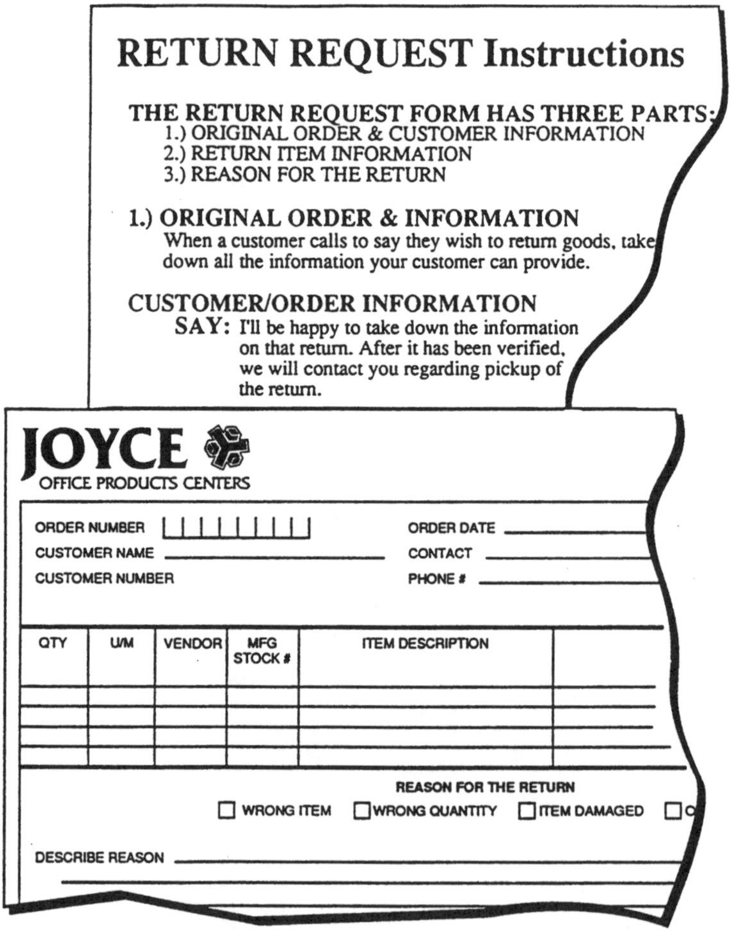

RETURN REQUEST Instructions

THE RETURN REQUEST FORM HAS THREE PARTS:
1.) ORIGINAL ORDER & CUSTOMER INFORMATION
2.) RETURN ITEM INFORMATION
3.) REASON FOR THE RETURN

1.) ORIGINAL ORDER & INFORMATION
When a customer calls to say they wish to return goods, take
down all the information your customer can provide.

CUSTOMER/ORDER INFORMATION
   SAY: I'll be happy to take down the information
              on that return. After it has been verified,
              we will contact you regarding pickup of
              the return.

JOYCE
OFFICE PRODUCTS CENTERS

| ORDER NUMBER | | | | | | | | | | ORDER DATE _____ |

CUSTOMER NAME _____   CONTACT _____

CUSTOMER NUMBER   PHONE # _____

QTY	U/M	VENDOR	MFG STOCK #	ITEM DESCRIPTION	

REASON FOR THE RETURN
☐ WRONG ITEM   ☐ WRONG QUANTITY   ☐ ITEM DAMAGED   ☐ O

DESCRIBE REASON _____

Finally, blueprints provide a mechanism for all parts of the organization to communicate and work together from a shared basis of understanding. The effort to build a blueprint in and of itself often is beneficial to companies in increasing knowledge of the total system among often separate departments and functions.

References

1. "Breaking Free from Product Marketing," *The Journal of Marketing*, (April 1977). Reprinted in *Services Marketing, Text, Cases & Readings*, Christopher Lovelock. (Englewood Cliffs, New Jersey: Prentice-Hall, 1984).

2. "How To Design a Service," in *Proceedings of the American Marketing Association* (Services Marketing Conference, Orlando, Florida 1981. Reprinted in the *European Journal of Marketing*, 16, no. 1, April 1982).

3. "Service Design in the Operating Environment," *Developing New Services: Proceedings of the 3rd Services Marketing Conference*, (Villanova University, Pennsylvania, October 1983). Edited by William R. George and Claudia R. Marshall. (Chicago: The American Marketing Association, April 1984).

4. "Designing Services That Deliver," *Harvard Business Review*, (January/February 1984). Reprinted in *Transformation of Banking* (Harvard University Printing Office, January 1984). Reprinted in "Implementing Marketing Strategies—Part II," *Harvard Business Review* (July/August 1984).

5. "Planning the Service Encounter," *The Service Encounter.* Edited by John A. Czepiel, Michael R. Solomon and Carol F. Surprenant (Lexington Books, January 1985).

6. "Service Positioning Through Structural Change," *The Journal of Marketing*, January 1987.

7. "How to Design a Service," in *The American Handbook of Marketing for the Services Industries.* Edited by Carole A. Congram and Margaret L. Friedman (Amacom, 1991).

8. "Understanding Services Through Blueprinting" *Advances in Services Marketing and Management—Research and Practice*, Vol. 1. Edited by Teresa A. Swartz, David E. Bowen and Stephen W. Brown, (JAI Press, Inc. in cooperation with The First Interstate Center For Services Marketing, Arizona State University, 1992).

Section IV
Marketing Channels and Selling Systems

The number of paths to the customer and the methods of selling to that customer have changed radically in the last generation. And those changes are only the beginning. As the articles in this section illustrate, the number of ways to reach one's customer will be limited only by one's imagination and the imaginative use of the tools available..

In "Channel Management 2000," John Mentzer explores the environmental changes and challenges that will make effective channel management critical to success in the next century. One of those newer channels, the wholesale distribution industry, is analyzed in depth by Adel el-Ansary. While the degree to which such organizations are wholesalers or retailers is open to debate, the impact they have had on the way all businesses operate and the critical nature of the challenges they face are indisputable.

Michael Czinkota explores similar relationships on a global scale in "Export/Import Marketing." The growing importance of global marketing is virtually unquestioned in today's world market, however, marketers often overlook the positive impact that effective global marketing can have on one's domestic efforts. Czinkota explains how greater knowledge of customers halfway around the world can contribute to success in one's own back yard.

Managing information as a way to reach customers effectively is the subject of Ken Bieschke's "List Management: What It Is, What It's Not," in which he explores how the information to be garnered from a company's "house list" can be an invaluable source of information and how its proper management can be the key to greater success and profits.

Marketers too often overlook the role of the direct salesperson in the marketing process. But the last four articles in this section, Gregg Baron ("Professional Selling for the Year 2000: Forces and Trends") and Tony Alessandra ("Collaborative Selling: The Future of the Sales Process") describe and analyze the forces and tools that are making the stereotypical "lone wolf" a truly extinct corporate species and will draw the sales professional of the future more closely to both the customer and to the organization. In "The Marketing Millennium Flowers," Bob Donath describes the new ways that business-to-business sales and marketing people will work with their customers. And in the concluding piece to this section, "Telemarketing," Steven F. Walker describes how the telemarketer of the future, using database technology, will dispel the negtive images of the past to become an essential part of the customer-focused, customer-driven marketing organization of the next century.

−18−
CHANNEL
MANAGEMENT 2000

John T. Mentzer

John T. Mentzer, Ph.D., is the Bruce Excellence Chair of Business Policy at the University of Tennessee Department of Marketing, Logistics, and Transportation, Knoxville. He has published in *Industrial Marketing Management, Journal of the Academy of Marketing Science, Columbia Journal of World Business, Research in Marketing, Journal of Business Logistics, International Journal of Physical Distribution and Logistics Management, Transportation and Logistics Review, Transportation Journal,* and other journals.

As we approach the year 2000, two prominent factors are shaping channel management: the growth in importance of international markets and rapid changes in the government regulatory environment. We will discuss these factors and then explore trends in channels to meet these environmental changes. Finally, we present a strategic planning perspective for channel management 2000.

Factors Shaping Channels

Although a number of factors affect channel management, we will focus on two major factors: the internationalization of markets and the changing government regulatory environment.

International Markets

Very few companies today have the luxury of defining their mission as a domestic corporation. Foreign suppliers, global communication technology, and foreign competition impact even companies that market their products solely within the borders of one country.

The cost and complexity of channel relations increase dramatically with international suppliers and customers. International suppliers often create a supply environment in which delivery times are quoted in terms of half a year, with order cycle variation measured in months. The production scheduling and inventory management implications of such long and variable lead times often negate the cost savings and supplier leverage advantages of international sourcing. The solution is to manage international supplier relations in such a way as to minimize lead time and its variability.

International customers also have unique and varied cultural preferences that complicate the channel management process. Cultural variations increase the probability of conflict in channel relations and complicate the process of channel flow.

Futurescope

There is growing evidence that channel relations will hold ever-increasing importance in the year 2000. For example, wholesaler-distributor sales are expected to grow faster than the economy throughout the entire decade of the 1990s.[1] Further, 76 percent of industrial goods manufacturers (traditionally thought to use direct means of distribution) use intermediaries/channels to distribute their products to the ultimate user.[2] Further, a number of environmental changes will create additional growth in the importance of channel management.

Such imperatives have increased the need for cross-cultural channel management initiatives that encompass the principles of multinational manufacturing and marketing, global inventory staging, and countertrade.

Government Regulatory Environment

Reregulation of a number of industries in many countries has created an environment in which the rules for managing channel relations is constantly changing. In just the past 15 years, managers have been confronted with major reregulation of the U.S. transportation, financial, and communications industries. In addition, such international initiatives as EC92 and NAFTA could have profound effects on the international environments of channel management.

It is incumbent on channel managers to develop flexible channel systems that survive and thrive in a constantly changing regulatory environment. Relationships that emphasize adaptability while still maintaining a value focus in the face of fundamental environmental changes are a challenge channel managers cannot ignore.

Channel Relationship Trends

The factors just discussed are and will continue to be driving forces for the major trends in channel relations.

Relationship Management

Relationship management (such as strategic alliances, supply chain management, and third-party arrangements) is a system of cooperative arrangements that transcend organizational boundaries to achieve channel goals. Innovative intermingling of business functions to achieve customer satisfaction is emphasized. Relationship management in essence forms a channel superorganization, with leadership typically provided by the member with the greatest risk. Central to such alliances is an understanding by all channel members of channel goals, roles of particular players, sharing of information, cross-organization functional shifting (e.g., marketing research, research and development, product design, and total system cost/value analysis), and a long-term commitment to the alliance. Thus, alliances solidly cement the long-term, cooperative channel relations orientation.

Information/Performance Emphasis

With the advent of powerful communications technology, channel managers have a wealth of information literally at their fingertips. This diffusion of information technology into channels is having a profound effect on how managers look at managing the channel.

Wide area networks, distributed data processing, individual personal computers, satellite communication systems, EDI, and a host of other information technologies have created an environment in which channel managers can mandate decentralized implementation of policies, while maintaining immediate centralized performance measurement over a myriad of activities.

The availability of detailed information significantly affects channel member relations. Performance measurement is considerably more accurate and timely, and thus corrective adjustment between members is more of an ongoing process. Further, conflict factors such as role ambiguity and differing perceptions of reality are reduced. In numerous channels, the advent of such technology has streamlined the channel and led to the elimination of some outside members, with enhanced communication and performance measurement allowing some channel functions to be absorbed by other channel members.

Service/Quality/Value-Driven Channels

Channels must be managed with the common focus on satisfaction of the final customer. This focus requires a cooperative effort to determine and effectively deliver the dimensions of the channel offering that are important to the customer.

Quality-driven channels demand research to understand the needs and requirements of customers, i.e., how customers define quality as it relates to their own satisfaction. Consequently, all channel members focus on delivering these needs and requirements every time. Quality-driven channels also demand communication, coordination, and cooperation from all personnel in the channel, regardless of organizational affiliation. As such, quality-driven channels raise the need for intimate channel relations to a higher level than in traditional channels.

In contrast to quality-driven channels, value-driven channels emphasize not just the delivery of the quality customers require, but also the guarantee that customers perceive the quality they are receiving. Thus, value-driven channels transcend a service/quality focus and require the delivery of quality and the delivery of the marketing of that quality to the customer as a vehicle for competitive advantage. Within this framework, the purpose of each channel member is to add value to the channel offering and/or provide communication of this value to the customer, i.e., to enhance perceived quality.

A Strategic Perspective

The preceding discussion has provided a perspective of the channel as a group of independent firms inextricably linked to accomplish goals that are increasingly tied to the concepts of information, performance, service, quality, and value. To manage these firms with these concepts as channel supergoals, a strategic perspective must be taken.

The strategic planning perspective is one in which organizations establish objectives that are consistent with a higher-order mission statement and define strategies to achieve each of those objectives.

Customer satisfaction will be the overriding mission of such coordinated, successful channels. This mission will encompass customer monitoring to determine those aspects of the channel delivery system that are important to the satisfaction of each customer and designing channel relationships and delivery systems to achieve those aspects.

This satisfaction mission will lead to the primary objective of the channel: to obtain value in all activities. Value-oriented channel management is an excellent tool for building closer relationships with key customers.

To achieve the objective of value attainment, all strategies must have as their underlying foundation a focus on quality and the control systems to monitor and maintain quality. The focus on quality must permeate the entire superorganization of the channel.

The channel can set itself apart from its competitors by efficiently delivering to customers those aspects they hold as important. It is the role of channel relations to establish and manage this process of efficient, effective delivery systems with the ultimate goal of strategic positional advantage in a dynamic environment.

Notes

1. Cespedes, Frank V., "Channel Management Is General Management," *California Management Review* (Fall 1988), 98–99.

2. "Mom and Pop Move Out of Wholesaling," *Business Week* (January 9, 1989), 91.

—19—
WHOLESALING
New Ways of Selling, New Forces and Challenges

Adel I. El-Ansary

Adel I. El-Ansary is the Eminent Scholar and first chairholder of the Paper and Plastics Education and Research (PAPER) Foundation Endowed Research Chair in Wholesaling at the College of Business Administration of the University of North Florida. In addition to his duties as Research Professor, he serves as Director of the Center for Research and Education in Wholesaling. He holds a Bachelor of Commerce degree from Cairo University, Cairo, Egypt, and an M.B.A. and Ph.D. from Ohio State University, Columbus, Ohio.

Because few people visit warehouses or are exposed to any purchasing transaction other than retailing, the wholesale distribution industry goes virtually unnoticed by the general public. However, the wholesale industry is a very large and diverse sector of the U.S. economy. Wholesale distribution accounts for approximately 10 percent of the national economic output, involves about 364,000 firms, employs 6.1 million persons, and sells an estimated $3.1 trillion in raw materials and manufactured products.

Defining the
Wholesale Distribution Industry

The Census Bureau categorizes wholesale trade in three ways: (1) manufacturers' sales branches, which sell direct; (2) agents and brokers, who sell manufacturers' goods but do not take title to them; and (3) merchant wholesaler-distributors, who take title and usually possession of goods for resale. Of the $3.1 trillion in goods that moved through wholesale trade in the United States, $1.8 trillion moved through wholesaler-distributors. In 1987, the last census of wholesale trade, merchant wholesaler-distributors accounted for 60 percent of the goods sold in the wholesale channel but 85 percent of the inventory being held. By the end of 1992, merchant wholesaler-distributors carried an estimated $205 billion in inventory.

The Merchant Wholesaler-Distributor

A merchant wholesaler-distributor is primarily engaged in purchasing goods from a supplier and selling those goods to another business. Some wholesaler-distributors manufacture products. Others sell a portion of their goods directly to consumers. Nevertheless, generally speaking, a wholesaler-distributor buys from a business and sells to a business. A wholesaler-distributor is providing a service—the right goods, at the right place, at the right time, at the right price—with

Futurescope

Warehouse clubs have emerged as a major force for creative revolution in the "retailing" industry. It is still not clear, however, how much of this business is really retailing and how much is wholesaling. Nevertheless, it will cause substantial changes in the way all other businesses operate. To become more competitive with wholesale clubs and supercenters, wholesaler-distributors' economic and operating models must be altered.

repackaging, technical assistance, help in marketing, financing, and other value-added services as required by customers.

The typical wholesale transaction involves a merchant wholesaler-distributor who takes title to goods supplied by others in the manufacturing, mining, agricultural, and wholesale sectors of the economy and resells them to others at a profit. Customers of wholesale establishments are mainly in the retailing, wholesaling, manufacturing, farming exporting, construction, commercial, and professional business sectors of the economy.

The sorting process is the key to economic viability of wholesalers. As channel intermediaries, they solve the problem of the discrepancy between various assortments of goods and services required by industrial and household consumers and the assortments available directly from individual producers. In other words, manufacturers usually produce a large quantity of a limited number of products, whereas consumers purchase only a few items of a large number of diverse products.

Wholesaler-distributors also participate in the performance of any or all of the marketing flows, that is, ownership, physical possession, promotion, financing, risk taking, negotiating, ordering, and payment. However, the rationale for wholesalers' existence boils down to the value-adding functions they perform for the suppliers and customers they serve.

The Wholesaler-Distributor Compared with the Manufacturer Direct

There are several reasons producers typically use wholesaler-distributors to get their products to market instead of selling direct themselves. A cost analysis of different distribution channels has shown that the cost of maintaining a manufacturer's branch office is significantly higher than the cost of using a merchant wholesaler. A wholesaler-distributor is often able to amortize the fixed costs of distribution over a broader product line than is typically handled by a single producer.

While manufacturers are more likely to be national or regional, wholesaler-distributors are closer to their markets geographically. Therefore, they largely assume the function of marketing, knowing where the local customers are and how to get at them.

Wholesaler-distributors also assume the cost of carrying inventory. Manufacturing tends to be a capital-intensive business, thus the use of wholesaler-distributors improves manufacturers' capital structure. Additionally, by holding inventory, wholesaler-distributors allow manufacturers to set efficient production schedules. Even though flexible manufacturing techniques are reducing product runs, most manufacturers have difficulty operating efficiently without the use of intermediaries to aggregate orders. Production also tends to require significant lead time.

Therefore, wholesaler-distributors shift the risk of market forecasting down the channel, allowing producers to concentrate on production.

The risk of bad debt is also assumed by the wholesaler-distributor. Local businesses are far superior to regional or national firms when it comes to assessing local credit risks, and assuming the function of trade credit improves the capital structure of manufacturing firms as well.

Finally, production and distribution seem to require different management skills. Production typically requires technical skills related to a specific product, whereas distribution is a service that requires the management of people.

Multiple Distribution Channels

The common perception is that goods go from a manufacturer to a wholesaler-distributor and then to a retail store, where they are purchased by consumers. In reality, the way goods move to market is more complicated. Products can go through the hands of several manufacturers and distributors and never even end up at a retail establishment. The end-user of these products can be a business, not a consumer.

Copper, for instance, can go through a series of transactions between several different manufacturers and wholesaler-distributors before it is finally purchased by the end-user as a component of another product. It can be sold from a metals producer to a metals wholesaler-distributor to a wire manufacturer to a wire wholesaler-distributor. The copper wire can next go to a motor manufacturer that sells its motors to an industrial distributor. The motor, with copper components, is then sold to a forklift manufacturer, which sells it to a materials handling distributor, where it is purchased finally by a woodworking shop. This example of a multiple distribution channel holds true for common consumer items sold in retail stores as well.

Economic Impact

Multiple wholesale distribution transactions contribute to the industry's size and importance to the economy. In 1992 there was approximately $3.1 trillion worth of goods that moved through wholesale trade in the United States, up an estimated 2.6 percent over the previous year. According to Census Bureau estimates, merchant wholesaler-distributors accounted for approximately $1.8 trillion of that total. In 1990 the gross domestic product was approximately 5.68 trillion "gross margin dollars." (Gross margin dollars measure the "value added," not sales.) Merchant wholesale-distribution generated 370 billion gross margin dollars in 1991. Therefore, merchant wholesale-distribution accounted for approximately 6.5 percent of total U.S. economic output.

Although the industry is highly fragmented, consisting of a few large companies and many small firms, merchant wholesaler-distributors are a critical source of jobs and income for communities throughout the nation. In 1991, merchant wholesaler-distributors employed about 4.6 million workers for whom compensation totaled more than $165 billion.

Although labor productivity in wholesale distribution in 1979 was well below the national average, one decade later it had risen to well above the national average. Just like the manufacturing sector in the 1980s, there was a "productivity explosion" in the wholesale distribution sector. Through advanced computer technology and new management practices, wholesale distribution firms have improved their productivity. The use of advanced computer systems has also improved inventory credit management, the selection of the most efficient channel of distribution, and market information flows. The benefits of these productivity gains can come in the form of higher margins for wholesaler-distributors or in the form of increased service or decreased prices passed on to the wholesaler-distributors' customers.

Strategies for Change

About 55 percent of all wholesale sales have been from the sale of products that have been in the market more than 5 years and are undifferentiated by quality. (In terms of 1992 sales figures, the most important merchant wholesale industries were groceries, machinery and equipment, and motor vehicles.) With the multitude of firms in wholesale markets all distributing products similar in quality, the competitive climate has become fierce.

Many wholesalers handling product lines are sensitive to changes in business conditions. Thus, they develop diversification strategies to increase sales and improve profit margins by minimizing sales fluctuations. Based on sales volume figures for 1990, some of the top wholesaling firms rely on both price and non-price competitive strategies to improve their margins.

Wholesalers with the shortest distance between them and their customers are generally more successful. To compete, therefore, many large wholesalers acquire or merge with other firms whose branches are in desirable locations, or they establish their own branches in order to locate as near as possible to a targeted market or valued customer. Other strategies are to increase the number of services provided with each product, to expand the number of product lines handled, and to concentrate on niche marketing.

–20–
EXPORT/IMPORT MARKETING
Lessons for Domestic Markets

Michael R. Czinkota

Michael R. Czinkota, Ph.D., is one of the nation's top international business and marketing experts. Serving as Deputy Assistant Secretary of Commerce during the Reagan Administration, Dr. Czinkota continues to advise government bodies and corporations on international trade, financing, and investment. A faculty member at Georgetown University, Dr. Czinkota publishes and is interviewed extensively in the trade press. He is a frequent and dynamic speaker on international issues.

Both exporting and importing constitute corporate efforts to expand the firm's market and resource base beyond the geographic and political limitations of the home market. As such, these activities are one step in the strategic direction of global marketing.

Benefits of Importing and Exporting

From a macro perspective, export and import activities determine the trade position of a country. A country needs to export in order to be able to afford imports of products and services that are either not available domestically or that improve the variety and quality of goods offered to its citizens. On the level of the firm, both exports and imports stimulate competitiveness. Furthermore, exports enable a more rapid movement on the learning curve through increases in production. As a result, the cost and price structure of the firm can be favorably affected.

On the import side, firms are able to obtain better or lower-cost sources of supply. This broadens the market offering and encourages other domestic firms to be more competitive in their activities. The end result is an increase in customer choice and the standard of living.

Reluctance of U.S. Companies to Export/Import

As a country, the United States under-exports. Estimates by the U.S. Department of Commerce indicate that one-half of all U.S. exports of manufactured products are made by only 100 companies, and that 80 percent of exports are made by 2,500 companies. Low U.S. participation in international trade is further evidenced by the comparatively low volume of U.S. per-capita exports. For example, in 1992

Futurescope

Successful exporting in the 21st century means that a firm can meet growing global competition head on and, in spite of transactional complexity, can profitably offer products that are in demand by foreign customers. In addition, the lessons learned from the export experience in areas such as product adaptation, cultural sensitivity, and competitive behavior can be applied to domestic activities and make the firm a more effective marketer back home.

Germany exported $5,370 a year for every man, woman, and child. The figure for the United States was only $1.750. Combined with a high propensity for imports, this export reluctance has resulted in a longstanding U.S. trade deficit, indicating that more is imported than is exported. This trade deficit in turn affects foreign investment, international indebtedness, and the value of the dollar.

Only about 100,000 U.S. firms are at least occasional exporters. The reluctance of so many U.S. business executives to seek overseas business opportunities has been attributed to the relative geographic isolation of the country and the large size of the domestic market. Before today's age of global linkages and interdependence, the U.S. economy was able to satisfy consumer wants and national needs with only minor reliance on international trade. Many executives still view exports as a marginal business and perceive exporting to be difficult to cope with, much too risky, and unprofitable. Due to the onslaught of international competition within the U.S. market, many executives have developed a fear of international activities. They tend to be unfamiliar with foreign market data resources and the international marketing assistance services that are available. As a result, they see only the risks—informational gaps, unfamiliar conditions in markets, and complicated domestic and foreign trade regulations—rather than the opportunities the international market can present. For example, firms that heavily depend on long production runs can increase their output dramatically by reaching customers abroad. Market saturation can be avoided by lengthening or rejuvenating product life cycles in other countries. Production policies that once were inflexible can now become variable when suppliers can be found on every continent. Overall, by participating in the global marketplace, firms can increase their profitbility and lower their risk.

Motivations to Export/Import

The export and import behavior and success of firms is related to managerial aspirations and the level of commitment that management is willing to give to the international effort. Because international markets cannot be penetrated overnight, and international sources of supply do not develop suddenly, there is a requirement for market development activity, market research, and sensitivity to foreign market factors. Only with long-term managerial commitment is the effort likely to be crowned by success.

Firms and their managers can either be proactive or reactive in their motivation to internationalize. Proactive motivations develop an internally generated strategic orientation and thrust by the firm. Main motivators are firm-specific advantages in the areas of cost structure, product uniqueness, or technology. Tax benefits and economy of scale considerations can also play a major role. Reactive motivations represent corporate responses to environmental pressures and changes. They consist of competitive pressures, declining domestic sales, overproduction, excess capacity, and saturated domestic markets. Typically, proactive firms are more likely to succeed internationally, because they enter the global market for the long term, rather than simply as a safety value or a back-up opportunity.

Once the decision to go international is made, firms tend to concentrate on markets of psychic proximity, which are markets that are geographically close and culturally similar to the home country. After gathering experience in these markets, firms then expand to more distant ones with a higher degree of comfort.

Stages of Entering Export/Import Activities

Even though some firms—particularly in smaller countries—are formed specifically to engage in international activities, in the United States firms tend to internationalize in a gradual fashion. After starting operations in the domestic market, over time some firms become involved in the global marketplace. This involvement appears to proceed in several distinct stages, in each one of which firms are measurably different in their capabilities, problems, and needs. First off, firms tend to become aware of international market opportunities yet do not take advantage of them. Later on, firms become interested and begin to accumulate information and investigate opportunities. As a next step, the firm executes some international transactions on a trial basis, which subsequently are evaluated as to their effectiveness and profitability. A negative assessment can result in a firm's renewed concentration on domestic market expansion. A positive evaluation, accompanied by a growth in the number of customers served and transactions carried out, will encourage a firm to adopt exporting and importing as a viable strategic option to be pursued and integrated with the overall corporate mission. Typically, this level is reached once international sales exceed 15 percent of sales volume. Over time, firms may then expand into additional or alternative international activities such as licensing, franchising, or direct foreign investment.

At the awareness level, firms are typically concerned and need help with operational matters such as information flows and the mechanics of carrying out international transactions. They understand that a totally new body of knowledge and expertise is needed and try to acquire it. Companies that have already had some exposure to international markets begin to think about tactical marketing issues such as communications and sales effort. Finally, firms that have reached the adaptation phase are mainly strategy and service oriented, worrying about longer-range issues such as service delivery and regulatory changes. In applying the marketing concept, one can recognize the increased sophistication of firms in international markets translates into a growing application of marketing knowledge. More exprience in international markets lets firms recognize that a marketing orientation is just as essential internationally as it is domestically.

Figure 1   A Model of the Export Development Process

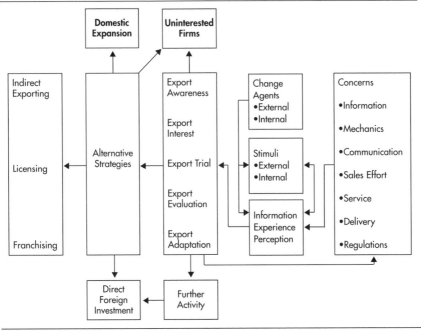

Source: Michael R. Czinkota and Ilkka A. Ronkainen, *International Marketing,* 3rd ed. (Fort Worth: Dryden Press, 1993), p. 261.

A model of internationalization, with a particular focus on exporting, is presented in Figure 1. It shows how the decision components combine into the export development process and how a firm gradually becomes an international player.

Government Encouragement of Exporting/Importing

To encourage the internationalization of firms, governments around the world engage in trade promotion. In rare instances, such promotion focuses on an enhancement of imports, particularly when governments feel strong pressure to reduce a bilateral or global trade surplus. More frequent are export promotion measures, which can yield tangible macro benefits such as job creation and an increase in the tax base. Governments conduct international negotiations to open foreign markets, remove obstacles to trade, or demand greater market access and foreign product acceptance abroad. On the level of the firm, export promotion aims to either decrease the risk or increase the profits. Government-support measures entail export counseling, information assistance, trade shows and trade fairs, export financing and insurance schemes, and preferential tax treatment. Increasingly, however, governments begin to recognize that the best export promotion consists of providing a domestic infrastructure and environment that enable firms to produce products and services that are globally competitive in quality and price and to offer them with international marketing expertise abroad.

For Further Reading

Michael R. Czinkota, *International Marketing Strategy* (Fort Worth: Dryden Press, 1994).

Michael R. Czinkota and Ilkka A. Ronkainen, *International Marketing,* 3rd ed. (Forth Worth: Dryden Press, 1993).

—21—
LIST MANAGEMENT
What It Is, What It's Not

Ken Bieschke

Ken Bieschke is President of Aggressive List Management, Inc., a full-service list and P.I.P. marketing/management firm dealing exclusively in areas related to the creation, maintenance, marketing, fulfillment, and accounting support of mailing list rental and package insert programs. He holds an B.B.A. degree from the University of Notre Dame and an M.B.A. from Northwestern Graduate School of Management, both in marketing.

List management is the popular term given to the practice of marketing mailing lists to direct marketing companies that use lists in making direct response solicitations. As such, the fundamental list management role is to promote the availability of a mailing list to a direct marketer that might rent the mailing list to use with a direct marketing mailing or telemarketing offer. It is termed a *rental* because the end-user of the list is generally entitled to a one-time use only, unless other terms are negotiated for multiple use or purchase of the list. This ensures that the owner of the list retains control and possession of the list. Rental requires the direct marketer to resubmit a request for use of the list whenever there is an interest in using it again.

The term *list management* is often confused with the closely tied functions of computerized list maintenance, a service that a list manager might or might not provide, but that is usually provided by outside computer houses called *service bureaus.* List maintenance services include list cleaning, editing, duplication removal, merging records, adding and deleting records, and data updates. List maintenance is essential to a list management program. It is the equivalent of a manufacturing function that provides the list manager with the finished product. Like any other manufactured product, quality control is critical, and it can vary from bureau to bureau.

List management is also sometimes confused with list brokerage, but they are in fact very different. List managers represent the list owner in the marketing effort of a list or lists. List brokers represent the list users (mailers or telemarketers) in

---

Futurescope

The list management function in the year 2000 and beyond will become more complex as the proliferation and subsegmentation of mailing lists continues to grow rapidly. The continued narrowing of consumer interests plays to the leading strength of direct marketing, which most cost-effectively targets marketing efforts to these special interests. The practices of list rental management are integral to the continued growth of direct marketing. List management professionals in the year 2000 and beyond must adapt to the sophistication that advanced computer technologies will have on the nature of lists. Databases will contain more information that managers will have to understand as their role as information managers continues to grow. Specialized knowledge beyond what list should work for what mailer's offer will be required of the list manager. List managers will have to know how to take advantage of technology to help direct marketers tap into mailing lists and databases so that they can market more cost-effectively.

the procurement of lists. There are typically four parties in every list rental transaction: list owner, list manager, list broker, and list user. In today's list marketing industry, most list rental transactions do include all four parties, particularly due to the value-added features managers and brokers bring to their respective clients, including in-depth knowledge about lists and list segments, what lists work and don't work for what mailers, who the influentials and decision makers are, how to negotiate special terms and pricing, and all of the concepts and theories developed that will help to maximize results in list usage.

It should be noted that because of the very similar nature of their functions, virtually all list brokerage businesses have list management divisions or affiliated businesses to serve both client sides, in recognition that most list users are also list owners, and vice versa. List management can be handled by the employees of a list owner or by an outside list management firm. Again, most list owners that rent out their lists have opted to employ the services of outside list management firms. There are approximately 200 list management firms in the United States today, as reported in the Standard Rate & Data Service (SRDS) publication *Direct Mail Lists—Rates and Data.* SRDS reports detailed information in this directory for approximately 50,000 business and consumer mailing lists currently available on the market for list rentals.

What a List Manager Does

A list manager has the responsibility to market a mailing list to parties (list brokers and/or mailers) that might want to rent the mailing list. Most list managers work on exclusive contractual agreements with their list owner clients and work on a commission arrangement.

The methodologies of a list manager in the list marketing function can include several media options, typically including direct mail, fax promoting, telemarketing, personal selling, trade show exhibiting, and space advertising.

Beyond the marketing function, a good list manager generally assumes several supporting responsibilities, including direct or indirect list maintenance and list rental fulfillment responsibility; accounting duties such as invoicing, collections, and remittances to list owners; and marketing analyses and reporting. List managers continually review and monitor the list user activity as well as outside market conditions and trends to be sure the list owner has a list product that has the greatest potential for attracting list renters.

Why List Managers Have Thrived

The outside list management industry is a relatively new one, springing forth only a few decades ago, and really taking form over the past 20 years. List management firms have thrived like most service organizations because they have specialized in a service field that their clients either cannot or prefer not to enter. In a service industry, the list management firm is steeped in the middle of information exchange and technology. The good list manager has both the computer support and decision-making influentials in its network that make its work the specialty of a full-time practitioner.

The list owner client that contracts a list manager derives all of the benefits of experience and expertise that the list manager can provide to a list marketing program. And the list owner can do so without any investment or ongoing expense, outside of the usual costs of list maintenance and fulfillment, because managers assume all expenses for the list marketing and support activities, including accounting and general administration.

Should You Rent Your List?

There are many factors that list owners must contemplate when evaluating whether to rent out their lists, but ten of the top positive benefits of renting can be summarized as follows:

Rental Profit

A list management program can be a lucrative profit center. For many list owners, it can produce as much or more than the sales of their products or services. Lists can have a wide range of value potential in list rentals, depending on many characteristics, but lists have been known to generate annual gross revenues from $.50 to $5 or more per name and address record. That means that a list of 100,000 records could produce annual rental revenues of $50,000–500,000. The average value of all lists seems to center around $1 per record, so the 100,000 record list would be worth $100,000. Again, that's just an average, and each list has its own unique value.

Positive Effect on Regular Business

Most list owners that rent out their lists find that their own offers to their lists generate better response rates. In theory, this is because the people on their lists are more active in direct-mail response, which makes them more prone to be responsive to multiple offers because they've had previous successful buying experiences.

Multi-Buyers Are the Best Customers

The more a customer has responded to offers historically, the more likely he or she is to do so in the future. Renting out lists makes more active customers of your own list.

Retaining Right of Refusal

List owners always retain the right to refuse or accept any request to rent their list, usually based on evaluating the nature and content of the offer from the prospective renter.

Security

Security measures have been invented that make list misuse a relatively rare event in the list rental transaction. List decoy or seeding systems have been developed that list users realize exist but are undetectable to everyone other than the list owner and manager. These techniques assure list owners that they can monitor all uses of the list.

Marketing Information

List owners have discovered they can learn much about their own lists just by sitting back and watching other firms that successfully use their list. An example is a crafts catalog company that finds that a jewelry merchandiser continuously rents its list. It may suggest a new product niche the craft company can open to the customer list it already owns. Reviewing the nature of the list users' offers can tell a list owner much more about the nature of its own list.

State of the Art

The direct marketing industry has evolved from the days when list owners were very protective of their lists . . . to the days when they would only make their lists available on mailing labels . . . to today's most common format of delivery being on magnetic tape. The R&D has been done over the past 25 years and strongly suggests to newcomers that there is a preponderance of benefits outweighing risks, based on the proliferation of lists made available for rentals.

Open Trade

List renting often benefits the list owner that wants to use another company's list, but would not be able to do so if it were not for its willingness to make its own list available reciprocally.

Lists Are Nonexclusive

There are some list owners that believe their lists are exclusively theirs, and if they don't rent them out, no one will be able to solicit their customers. The reality is that those same customers are most likely included on one or more other lists and are being reached with solicitation from other companies.

Easy Entry and Exit

A list owner can easily get into and out of a list management program. There are no heavy capital investment or inventory requirements. A list owner can test the waters and quickly determine whether the benefits outweigh any negative impact of a list rental program.

Trends Toward the Year 2000

Computerization has been the most significant contributor to the explosion of list renting. Through computerization, the merging and purging of millions of names and addresses can be completed in a few hours. Lists can be segmented with specific data that in effect create many lists within lists and allow renters to find responsive subsegments of a list that they can mail to successfully.

Today and toward the year 2000, list owners and mailers are continuing to seek methods that make it possible to enhance their chances of making successful direct response offers. Mailing lists that historically contained only names and addresses are now being expanded to include more demographic and buying behavior information that helps to target future marketing efforts.

The narrow focus that such database identification processes allow is analogous to the same evolution of niche marketing that we have seen in other media. For example, mass magazine and general television broadcasting evolved to specialty magazines and special-interest cable programming. It is fitting that direct marketing continues to innovate in this role, because more than any other marketing method, direct marketing was the first to recognize the importance of class versus mass marketing.

Concerns for the Future

Like any industry, list management and direct marketing in general have concerns that will need to be addressed more vigorously was we proceed to the year 2000 and beyond. A growing public concern about privacy, security, and the environment places much demand on the list user community to be sensitive to public opinion. Direct marketing companies and their associations must educate the public on the benefits served by an ongoing direct marketing industry that includes the renting of lists, that allows these companies to grow, and also benefits the recipients who want to receive their offers. The outlook for direct marketing is that it still has much potential for growth. List management will have a continued fundamental role to play in supporting this ongoing development.

—22—
PROFESSIONAL SELLING FOR THE YEAR 2000
Forces and Trends

Gregg Baron

Gregg Baron is a Certified Management Consultant with extensive experience in the areas of customer service, team building, sales development, collaboration, executive coaching, and NeuroLinguistic Programming (NLP). As Founder and President of Success Sciences, he has developed his expertise through working with a wide variety of organizations including Motorola, USA Today, Florida Power, Sony, Pioneer, IBM, Continental Airlines, and Novell. He is the author of *The Idea-A-Day Guide to Super Selling and Customer Service,* as well as numerous articles in professional journals.

Sales professionals need to be students of change. They need to focus on, respond to, and anticipate changes that new technology will bring. Technological changes that affect a customer's business should be a consideration in approaching your customers, regardless of what you sell.

Sales Trends

Specific macro trends that customers expect, and how a sales organization can respond proactively, ultimately touch what sales professionals must do to differentiate themselves and be effective in the future. These macro trends include technology, service guarantees, customization, timeliness, security of data, and collaboration. Critical to this effort and payoff is anticipation of needed action versus reaction to events when it is too late. And the time to build a bridge to the next paradigm is now, while your existing paradigm still works.

Technology

Technology is the base trend that affects the trends to follow. Changes in technology have changed competition, the sizes of companies, life-styles, expectations, communication, presentations, and virtually everything else.

Sales professionals will continue to be affected by sales technology shifts in their and their customers' industries. Sales technology shifts, such as overnight shipping, video teleconferences, mobile communication, laptop computers, and the like, will affect them and their competitors. These shifts for salespeople and their customers can become competitive advantages when appropriately acted on. The only option is to align with and make use of the multiple levels of change driven by the creation and application of technology—or simply lose out.

Unconditional Service Guarantees

A recent statistic indicated that people are now changing jobs an average of once every three years. In addition, the proliferation of restructuring or "rightsizing" goes on with no end in sight. With these layoffs and voluntary job changes, the people on the purchasing side of the business-to-business transaction are under more pressure than ever. They have more responsibility and less time as they juggle multiple items in multiple areas, some of which they are not experts in. With that juggling comes a need to know—without looking over a vendor's shoulder—that the products and services they purchased will be delivered exactly as promised. The expectation of a hassle-free relationship has grown from the very real need for such a relationship.

Unconditional service guarantees respond to the changes in the way people do business and their expectations for quality and reliability. In the sales encounter, there is a continuum of perceived financial and psychological risk for the buyer. These perceived risks are highest when the relationship is new, the expense is

Futurescope

Need evidence that the world is changing dramatically? Just pick up a newspaper. There are changes involving nearly every aspect of our lives—from dramatic political shifts such as the fall of communism in Europe, to new technologies, to shifts in the way people relate to one another (e.g., 30 years ago, "significant others" were spouses). These changes and others are reflected in the day-to-day business world and sales professionals need to be aware of them and anticipate their impact as they move into the new century.

substantial, and the transaction is linked to things considered vital to the buying organization. Unconditional service guarantees are an important strategy for managing that perceived risk because, at least in theory, they eliminate that risk. Unconditional service guarantees are, without a doubt, linked to the new realities in the marketplace. It is one strategy that, at the moment, will differentiate you. However, in the future, it will become commonplace and therefore add no differentiation.

Customization

People want flexibility, choice, and involvement when buying solutions. Customers have become more demanding and increasingly are expressing unique requirements. When these requirements can be fulfilled, they add value to the relationship. Adding customization to what you sell delivers on those needs because it adds a sense of control for the buyer. The trend of more and more providers of products and services focusing on customization as a differentiator is undeniable. It has extremely powerful sales benefits, especially when it leads to saving customers time, effort, or money by providing exactly what they want without having to make compromises when choosing to do business with you.

Time

Time is money. Changes in technology, customer expectations, and competition have enabled the production of high-quality, often customized goods to be delivered in increasingly shorter time frames. Customer expectations continue to increase as competitors raise the bar on quality and value. Value can be enhanced by quality, service, added features, price reduction, customization, or reduction of time.

The increased importance of time-based competition can be seen when looking at a couple of dramatic changes. Explore the history of how people have purchased food and how that has changed dramatically over the years. We progressed from buying supplies at the general store, to traditional restaurants, to fast-food restaurants.

Time-based competition and the need to shrink the time between the decision to by and the delivery of products or services is evident in how we communicate with people in our personal lives.

In less than 200 years we have gone from sending written communication via Pony Express, to trains, to telegraph, to overnight delivery, faxes, mobile faxes, online electronic billboards, and E-mail. We now have video telecommunication systems that change when, where, and how we can do business. We now shop from catalogs and TV shopping channels that enable us to call, order, and conclude a product transaction in minutes, with next-day delivery commonplace.

The shift toward near-instantaneous communication and response affects how we live, how we want to live, and how we do business. It also affects our selling strategies and tactics, including mobile communications such as working on airplanes, cars, and trains with cellular and other mobile communication technology; faxing documents and placing equipment inside a client's organization that puts them online to our services for ordering and maintenance. The demand for the delivery of high-quality, customized goods and services in a fraction of the time that used to be acceptable is a reality today. Fulfilling that demand is an opportunity for selling in the future.

Security of Data

Information is increasingly becoming the currency of choice. Information, whether it is a proprietary industrial process or the intimate details of our personal credit, income, savings, travel, and spending patterns, also is sensitive. People around the world have a high level of concern for the security of their data. Transactions need to be designed to manage the perceived financial and psychological risks associated with customer information. More and more business clients are requiring confidentiality agreements before doing business. The sales professional's effectiveness depends on anticipating the level of those concerns and creating the appropriate strategy for dealing with them. This trend and the final trend that will be discussed are relationship issues.

Collaboration

Fierce competitors such as Apple and IBM have begun to share technology and to collaborate on research and development. This stunning example of corporate collaboration works down to the micro level within high-performance organizations that organize diverse departments to work together in cooperative, unified efforts to achieve common goals. This spirit also reaches down to individuals who have increasingly high levels of narrowly focused expertise and whose value consists of having the ability to collaborate with other highly expert people in other areas. It begins with a shared understanding of the outcome and the process for getting there. Collaboration speaks specifically to joint ownership and involvement for both "the what" and "the how" of working with others.

The Sales Equation of Tomorrow

Sales success in the future can be summarized in the following equation: Technology × Collaboration = Unconditional service guarantees + Customization + Data security + Time-based competition.

Why this equation? The most dramatic force for change in our lives has been technological change. Several brief examples were given previously, but here is an example form one life: President Harry S Truman was born in 1884, when the fastest from of multidirectional transportation was the horse—at approximately 8 miles per hour. He was 19 years old, the age of the average college sophomore, when the Wright brothers flew the first aircraft in 1903. As U.S. president, he authorized the dropping of the first atomic bomb in 1945, and he was still alive when the first human being set foot on the moon in 1969.

Today's rate of change is virtually unparalleled in human history, and the only way that business will survive, much less prosper, is through collaboration with both customers and colleagues to a greater extent and more intensely than ever. The product of that collaboration will be products and services that are unconditionally guaranteed, are customized to a specific customer's needs, provided at a faster rate than imagined only a few years ago, and done with the customer's needs for security and confidentiality respected and assured.

At the center of this will be the new sales professionals. They need to shift to collaborating with the other salespeople in their organization to create competitive advantages in strategy and skill by sharing their knowledge about products, markets, clients, and patterns. They also should collaborate with the non-sales professionals in their organization to provide higher efficiencies in meeting unique customer needs for reliability, responsiveness, and relationships. The sales professional of tomorrow will work to build successful collaborative customer relationships that create extraordinary leverage through new levels of loyalty that result in repeat and referral business. Successful sales professionals of tomorrow will align with these trends today and differentiate themselves accordingly.

—23—
COLLABORATIVE SELLING

The Future of the Sales Process

Tony Alessandra

Tony Alessandra, Ph.D., is a leading sales speaker and trainer based in La Jolla, California. He has authored numerous books, audio, and video programs, including *Collaborative Selling, Idea-a-Day Guide to Super Selling,* and *The Competitive Advantage.*

There are several reasons for the dramatic changes that have taken place in the marketplace and in the nature of the sales process. These sources of change include new technologies, globalization, too many choices in the market, and sophisticated buyers. No doubt you have seen this quantum shift and its consequences in your industry: your competitors have increased in number and become more aggressive. Your products or services are more difficult to sell than in the past. It has become a challenge just to differentiate your company from your competitors, and price issues are a constant problem.

Technology

For most products and services, technology is available to virtually everyone; if not today, then tomorrow. In the past, it was possible to develop a technology that would give a company a competitive advantage for a couple of years. Now, however, technological advantages are so shortlived that their ability to differentiate the company is fleeting, at best. Only a few dominant companies can claim that their product is radically different for very long. It does not matter whether you are selling consumer electronics (especially computers), furniture, cars, or copy machines. Every manufacturer has access to the same technology and, therefore, offers the same product features.

The Global Market

We are now in a global economy that affects every company. There are more and different competitors than in the past, and they have helped create a confusion in the marketplace, not only for corporate executives, but also for their customers.

Futurescope

The world of business has changed—and continues to change—dramatically and rapidly. Markets have grown from local to national to global. Technology no longer offers a competitive advantage, and customers have become much more savvy. All of these changes and more have created an environment in which salespeople must adopt new attitudes, learn new skills, and gain a new understanding of how to approach their markets and work with customers.

Supply Exceeds Demands

For most products and services in most parts of the world, supply exceeds demand. Customers today are experiencing over-choice, a phenomenon that was described first by Alvin Toffler in his seminal book *Future Shock*. Over-choice is a stressful state caused by too many choices. Buyers are overwhelmed with more choices of products and suppliers than they could ever possibly use.

Sophisticated Buyers

The positive side of over-choice is that it has created a world full of sophisticated, well-informed consumers. People are more willing to (1) research their options, (2) slow down the decision-making process, and (3) insist on doing business with companies and salespeople whom they like.

The upshot of these market influences is that the differentiated products of yesterday are the commodities of today. Instead of making differentiation easier, technology has made differentiation more difficult. Differentiation is, however, the only way to be successful in today's market. Differentiation must come from quality, price, or service, and few companies can survive competing on price. This is a monumental challenge that every company faces. It is a challenge met by collaborative selling, a system in which salespeople can create differentiation—and its accompanying competitive advantage—every time they go after business.

The Fallacy of Traditional Selling Techniques

The traditional approach to selling was largely developed after World War II. When the war ended, the demand for consumer goods shot up to an all-time high. Consumers were not very sophisticated, so selling techniques revolved around the following scenario, which still exists today.

Traditional salespeople paid little attention to targeting their markets or planning their sales calls. They approached the market as a "numbers game" and delivered a canned pitch to as many prospects as possible in the shortest amount of time. Good salespeople began by breaking the ice with a little small talk (and equated small talk with relationship building). Then they delivered razzle-dazzle pitches to wide-eyed prospects, whom they hoped were receptive. There was little, if any, information gathering. Instead, the sales process focused on a persuasive pitch, manipulative closing techniques, and the salespeople were those who had mastered the art of arm-twisting.

This traditional sales pitch was, by necessity, generic. All of the product's features and benefits had to be covered, because salespeople had no way of knowing which features and benefits were relevant. It was a true shotgun approach in which salespeople tried to sell their products to every prospect, regardless of need. There was no follow-up after the sale. Traditional salespeople moved from one transaction to the next without looking back. Sales were perceived as one-shot deals.

Traditional selling is not dead. It is still used in the automobile industry. Despite the changes in the marketplace and their desperate need for differentiation, many car dealers are still insulting their customers with high-pressure, traditional tactics. They are short-term thinkers who must assume there is an endless supply of new customers.

Is this the basis for long-term relationships? Is this the formula for success? Certainly not. General Motors had its worst year in its history in 1992. In November 1993, an article in the *Wall Street Journal* reported that Chevrolet had just woken up and was making customer satisfaction the focus of a full-scale makeover effort. Why so late? Companies such as Nordstrom, L.L. Bean, Federal Express, and others discovered and implemented that years earlier.

Traditional selling has another Achilles' heel. It created tension and can be construed as adversarial. Traditional salespeople often perceive their prospects as people with whom they must go to battle to win business. This power-struggle mindset is supported by sales trainers who teach manipulative sales techniques and by books with combative titles such as *Hard Ball Selling, Guerrilla Marketing,* and *The Sale Begins When the Customer Says No.*

It does not take a genius to realize that the focus in traditional selling is misplaced and myopic. The commando approach to selling is obsolete. It does not foster referrals, references, repeat business, word-of-mouth advertising, customer satisfaction, or goodwill.

Collaborative Selling

Collaborative selling begins with a different mindset: a commitment to the long term. Today's customers buy differently, so today's salespeople must sell differently. Customers know there is no urgency to buy, because good deals, good salespeople, and good companies come along every day. Price is less of an issue, because buyers are not just interested in great deals; they want great relationships. Today's customers are looking for measurable quality in the products and services they buy.

The transition to collaborative selling and the emphasis on long-term relationships is evident in the words and phrases used to describe modern buyer-seller relationships: strategic alliances, sustaining resources, single resources, integrity, values, and ethics.

Today's customers are looking for long-term relationships with suppliers who will be reliable resources over the long haul. In fact, many companies are awarding lifetime contracts to their supplier-partners. Collaborating companies are networking their computer systems to expedite order-entry, just-in-time inventory control, and electronic payment. Strategic alliance, partnering, collaboration—call it what you will—is taking place throughout the world on a macro level (industry to industry) and on a micro level (salesperson to customer).

Collaborative selling means handling every aspect of the sales process with a high degree of professionalism. There are six basic steps that describe how the collaborative sales process unfolds: target, contact, explore, collaborate, confirm, and assure.

Target

The first step is a marketing necessity: understand exactly what the product/service is and identify the specific markets that can best use it. This is done on a company level in the marketing plan and should be done by individual salespeople as well. It takes some time, but careful planning focuses effort and provides a greater return on time and money invested. Collaborative salespeople know they must concentrate on prospects who have a high probability of buying.

Contact

The first step after targeting a market is to contact customers in a cost-effective and professional way. Naturally, this would be some combination of letter, phone, and personal contact. The right combination of contacting strategies ensures that collaborative salespeople create high perceived value before they call on their prospects.

When contact is made, collaborative salespeople set the stage for a cooperative working relationship. They convey their desire to explore needs and opportunities. They build credibility and trust. They express their sincere desire to be of service, and they make their competitive advantages known without jumping into a presentation.

Explore

In this stage of the collaborative sales process, salespeople convey the message: "Let's explore your business situation to see if there are needs to fulfill or opportunities on which to capitalize."

During the explore stage, collaborative salespeople conduct research, meet with their prospects frequently, and do whatever it takes to become an expert on their prospect's business. The give-and-take relationship that develops sets the stage for in-depth exploration of options that might culminate in a sale. Collaborative salespeople make it clear that they want to help, not just make a sale. If, after information gathering, collaborative salespeople find that their products are not appropriate for their prospects, which is unlikely due to their careful target marketing, they will forego the sale but will have made a friend and business contact.

Collaborate

It is at this point, after an in-depth exploration of a prospect's situation, that collaborative salespeople talk about their products or services. Naturally, they are discussed in the context of the prospects' needs or opportunities.

Collaborative salespeople never dictate solutions to their prospects. Instead, they form "partnerships" in which prospects play an active role in the search for the best solutions. The collaborate phase of the sale is conducted in the spirit of "let's work together on the solution and together build a commitment to its successful implementation." This team approach to problem solving ensures that prospects will be committed to solutions. by making customers equal partners in problem solving, collaborative selling reduces or eliminates the risk inherent in the customer's decision-making process.

Confirm

Keep in mind that, in every phase of the collaborative selling process, the salesperson and prospect have communicated well. Collaborative salespeople move on to the next phase of the sales process only after they have received assurances that their customers are in agreement with them on everything that has been discussed.

This agree-as-you-go process eliminates the need to "close" the sale or handle objections. Most objections have surfaced long before this point. If resistance does occur, the salesperson simply gathers more information or clarifies a detail.

With collaborative selling, the sale is a matter of when, not if. Confirming the sale is the logical conclusion to an ongoing communication and problem-solving process. There is no need to "close" them. People commit when all their buying criteria are met!

Assure

This phase of the collaborative sales process begins immediately after the sale has been confirmed. Collaborative salespeople keep in touch after the sale. They communicate regularly about delivery dates, installation, training, and other relevant matters. They make sure their customers are satisfied with their purchases. They help customers track their results and analyze the effectiveness of the solution.

Collaborative selling is the key to differentiation on the micro level. It represents an obsession with quality and customer satisfaction. It reflects a high degree of professionalism and a primary focus on relationships rather than transactions. It is clear that collaborative selling is a mutual-win situation, one that provides increased security to both parties. This increased security is exactly what customers want and need, given the market changes that are occurring so rapidly.

Collaborative selling is a philosophy and practice being used today by enlightened salespeople, and it is clearly the sales process of the future. Collaborative selling helps professional salespeople build large, loyal customer bases that generate future sales, provide referrals, and act as lifetime annuities.

The Future of Selling and Salespeople

Collaborative salespeople of the future will gain a tremendous competitive advantage from PC technology. Computer software programs will become salespeople's smart assistants on the road and in the office.

Imagine a software program called "Collaborative Selling." This program would combine the time-efficiency functions of a contact management program with the coaching and training of a full-time sales trainer. The program would help the salesperson in each phase of the sales process. In the target phase, the computer would be used to help keep the prospect pipeline full. Direct-mail letters could be generated on a predetermined schedule. Phone calls could be scheduled (and the individual reminded) automatically.

During the contact phase, salespeople could talk on the phone and be coached by the computer simultaneously. Did you forget a competitive advantage statement? Click on an icon and a half-dozen statements appear. Want to know how to respond to some common brush-offs? Click on another icon and the answers to the most common initial resistance appear.

The concept of the computer as coach has tremendous potential. The smart software of the future will be able to take a sales philosophy such as collaborative selling, combine it with a personality system such as People Smart (similar to Carlson Learning's DISC system or Wilson Learning's Social Styles), and mix them with a contact management program that will serve as secretary and coach. The program would ask about the prospect's personality style: Is she a director, socializer, relater, or thinker? Don't know? The computer will show you how to find out. Need some tips on the best way to approach a director in the explore phase of the sale? The computer will coach you. Need to send a letter to a socializer in the contact phase of the sale? The computer will automatically select letters that relate to that phase of the sale and the prospect's personality style.

Smart, interactive software holds great promise for collaborative salespeople. Prospecting and target marketing will become streamlined and more accurate. Relationship building will become faster and easier. Contacting will become more sophisticated and effective. Penetrating current accounts and getting referrals will be more fruitful.

Salespeople of the future might use traditional PCs, or they might use laptops, or they might do the majority of their business by teleconferencing. Or they might use some other form of technology not even imagined today. The rate and direction of change in computer technology has been so rapid that most sensible prognosticators want to temper or qualify their predictions about technology in the future. But one thing is certain: whatever tools salespeople are armed with, they will use them to craft mutually beneficial relationships that will advance the objectives of themselves, their companies, and their clients for the long term.

—24—
BUSINESS MARKETING 2000
The Marketing
Millennium Flowers

Bob Donath

Bob Donath is a well-known speaker and author on the subjects of business-to-business advertising and marketing. His career represents a unique combination of experience and accomplishment in the fields of publishing, journalism, and marketing management. Mr. Donath now heads his own marketing and marketing communications consulting firm, Bob Donath & Co., in White Plains, New York, specializing in business-to-business marketing. His clients include marketing services firms, corporate marketing communications departments, and a business-academic think tank at a major university. He is the co-author of *Managing Sales Leads: How to Turn Every Prospect into a Customer,* and is a regularly featured columnist in the American Marketing Association's *Marketing News* newspaper. Mr. Donath holds a master's degree in marketing from Northwestern University's Kellogg School of Management, and a bachelor's degree from Northwestern's Medill School of Journalism.

Nearing the close of the 20th century, business buying accounted for roughly $7 of every $11 in U.S. goods and service purchases, yet its importance remains largely hidden from public view. Business marketing has been the traditional also-ran in the view of the public and the marketing profession alike. The glamorous and ubiquitous advertising and massive budgets characterizing consumer marketing campaigns command nearly all the attention the press and the college classroom devote to the marketing subject. Because everyone is a prospect, consumer product and service marketing stand out by several orders of magnitude.

Adding to the insult, business marketing also has suffered a back-seat status in its own habitat. Traditionally, account-oriented industrial firms concentrate sales force effort on individual accounts and distributors. In conventional manufacturing thinking, marketing has been a sales support function rather than the strategic umbrella for the selling effort. Even worse, companies struggling to maintain competitive advantages through technology perceive marketing as a technically oriented function, much closer to the R&D lab than to customers.

By the year 2000 or shortly thereafter, the marketing concept will have flowered, finally, in many industries. Ironically, marketing as we know it today could disappear as a distinct function with its own box on the corporate organization chart.

The Information That Counts

Strategic lessons learned the hard way fueled much of the prominent business news in the early 1990s. Firms recovering from the speculative binges of the 1980s made "reengineering" to concentrate on "core competencies" their war cry. Among the

Futurescope

The best days for the business marketing function lie ahead, but getting there won't be half the fun. To prosper in the next millenium, companies serving business customers will face major changes in the way they go to market. Current trends have eroded the established role of marketing in the industrial firm, pushing it to the forefront of corporate business strategy. By the mid 1990s, the time of this writing, down-sized corporate staffs, leaner marketing budgets, global marketplaces, and parsimonious buyers forced smarter firms to adopt new tools for battling price erosion, channel discord, foreign competition, and finicky customers. The future suggests that companies hewing to the traditional model in years to come won't be around to see how it all turns out in the 21st century.

prominent lessons was IBM's wrenching restructuring, overcoming what had been too much emphasis on maintaining an outdated status quo. Another 1980s computer industry icon, Digital Equipment Corp., struggled through its own epiphany, learning to market solutions rather than sell technology. The tough lessons weren't the computer industry's alone, of course; slow growth and market change outpacing marketing skills stung all business marketers to varying degrees.

To see the future, however, look beyond the hyperbole of popular buzzwords such as "paradigm shifts," "customer satisfaction," "virtual corporations," and "strategic alliances," to name but a few. There one finds marketers fashioning new ways of harnessing information of the most critical type: knowledge of the customer. Using advanced research, modeling, and database tools, successful marketers on both the consumer and industrial sides of the business capture competitive advantage from knowing, simply, what individual customers want. No longer is the buyer a faceless mass of consumers or some mass-market statistical model deriving abstract market niches. The customer, to use the phrase popularized by the Boston Consulting Group, is a "segment of one." The impact that will have on marketing and all other functions in the firm in the 21st century will be profound.

Yes, salespeople always worked with individual account-by-account information in business markets. But they didn't have enough of it, nor did their corporate employers collect and exploit the information fully to control the entire company's response to the marketplace, from R&D through engineering, manufacturing, procurement, finance, and personnel. When the marketing concept finally becomes the prime driver of business and industrial corporate strategy, customer-oriented information will tie every employee in every function of the company to the goals of the marketing strategy. In effect, all will become marketers.

Response to Needs

Perhaps because it is so self-evident, traditional marketing organizations have seemed to forget on occasion that customers behave only to their own advantage. The tighter the fit between the individual buyer's needs and the product or service offering, the more competitive the offering. Recognizing that, firms have rushed to embrace the tools of total quality management (TQM) for maximizing customer-perceived value. But as manufacturing technologies and customer needs-assessment techniques improve, the TQM imperative to "do the important things right" still will not be enough. The 21st-century solution, the gurus predict, lies in corporate "agility."

The "agile enterprise," a grand objective promoted by the Agile Manufacturing Enterprise Forum (AMEF) at Lehigh University's Iacocca Institute, promises genuinely exciting times for marketing people. Nominally, agility looks to the production function. Yet it is really about serving markets, the company becoming one fully integrated engine of customer satisfaction. Dysfunctional interdepartmental corporate barriers will fall, and the engineer and marketer will become soul brothers, goes the agility catechism. It is the natural culmination of all quality-orientation movements of today, proclaim the blue-chip corporate, academic, and consulting experts at AMEF.

Contraction and Resolution

As the old saw goes, "People don't buy electric drills. They buy holes." Therefore, according to a tenet of the marketing concept, customers do not buy products. They buy solutions. Manufacturing agility becomes the embodiment of genuine market orientation.

Yet the promise of turn-on-a-dime customization of technology to fit each customer's need exactly contains a basic contradiction. Can a manufacturer be both an agile marketer and a competitive technologist? The answer will appear in the corporate reengineering dramas of the 1990s. However, it may well be "no."

The intellectual and cash investments advanced basic technologies require make them ever more sluggish obstacles to market dexterity. That's acceptable in markets where technical superiority is an overarching success factor. But competitors and scientific advances quickly undermine that advantage as today's breakthrough becomes tomorrow's ho-hum commodity. All the early 1990s talk of "agility" in the United States and "holonics" in Japan contemplates improved manufacturing technologies mitigating that vicious cycle. However, by the time of this writing, those notions were theoretical rather than demonstrable in practice.

Meanwhile, the firms best sustaining market presence with end-users will be those integrating whatever technologies it takes, from whatever sources, to maximize value to the customer. They will be the ultimate embodiment of agile marketing, not actually "making" anything physical themselves, but cobbling others' products into services that solve customer problems. In a sense, it's the classic original equipment manufacturer role expressed to the nth degree.

Driven by those forces, business markets will transform from today's vertical orientation to interlaced webs of technologist producers exchanging goods and intellectual capital (the customer solutions) among themselves. The demand for integrated solutions combining several technologists' capabilities will foster a variety of alliances among producers: not necessarily the long-term supplier-buyer marriages hailed in the 1990s concept of strategic alliances—quickly shifting competition will not allow such rigidity—but quickly made, opportunistic responses to individual customers' unique needs. When mutually advantageous, even erstwhile competitors will team up to snare a particular market niche opportunity.

High-tech marketing expert William Davidow labeled such arrangements the creation of virtual corporations, adapting the computer engineering concept of virtual entities. Prolific joint venture formation among electronics, computer, and communications firms in the mid-1990s already are bringing the virtual corporation notion to life. The drive to achieve market credibility through the standards-setting process creates a blizzard of technology-sharing declarations. Even celebrated rivals such as IBM and Apple Computer, and Microsoft and Novell, attempt to cooperate, at least publicly, in pursuing future niches while continuing to brutalize each other in their bread-and-butter markets.

Long Road to Nirvana

Getting there will not be easy. Some of today's trends might be moving corporate strategies in the wrong direction.

One dysfunctional craze is the uncritical acceptance of customer satisfaction as the key marketing yardstick. By the early 1990s, more than 160 research firms claimed expertise in customer satisfaction surveys, according to one count. Survey results increasingly have become part of marketing managers' compensation algorithms at leading-edge firms. Not that satisfying customers isn't important, but making satisfaction an explicit objective risks misunderstanding what's really happening in the marketplace.

The term *satisfaction* implies that one has reached an absolute level of customer acceptance where everything is hunky-dory, peachy-keen, and swell. The customer gets everything he or she desires. Some add a semantic twist and declare that "customer delight" or the "thrilled customer" is the noblest, most important goal. Whatever the rhetoric, attaining satisfaction requires the firm to provide "satisfactory" performance on all dimensions, beefing up its weaknesses as well as maintaining its strengths. Palpable weakness performing any of the various tasks demanded by the customer means the customer isn't yet "satisfied."

That prescription could, however, lead to disaster. Instead of squandering its inevitably finite resources attempting to bolster every facet of its offering, the firm should ensure that competitors cannot match its strengths, the virtues that won it customers in the first place. It matters less that the customer feels some sort of warm glow of gruntlement, than the firm do the important things better than rival vendors to win and keep the business.

Also, measuring satisfaction by surveying current customers doesn't explain why non-customers buy from someone else. Segment-by-segment key-factor analysis is the better research objective, making sure that opportunities that could be exploited but as yet aren't are not overlooked.

Finally, is it reasonable to expect that even satisfied customers will admit their joy? It's not likely, as any salesperson who has had to negotiate a price quickly learns. Acknowledging contentedness vitiates a buyer's ability to wangle a price concession or other favor out of the seller. As marketing professor Irwin Gross of the Pennsylvania State University points out, negotiation really hinges on the relative value each party wins. How much of the transaction's total value does the buyer capture by extracting price and/or service and terms concessions? How much does the seller win by making price premiums stick?

A better marketing metric than customer satisfaction might simply be growth in the firm's share of customer purchases, the Boston Consulting Group's David Edelman has argued. Objective and relatively easy to determine, the share yardstick focuses the supplier organization on improving customer service even more, obviating the organizational complacency that sets in when "satisfaction" has been achieved.

Ties That Bind

Long-term vendor-supplier alliances—some so cozy they resemble vertical integration—became fashionable in word if not always in deed during the 1980s. Uncertain markets and complex technologies encouraged experimentation with relationships other than the traditional selling strategy of transaction-oriented adversarial dealings. Suppliers and buyers alike found that nurturing lasting alliances with key customers outweighed any need for flexibility. In many cases, buyers rather than suppliers demand close collaboration, recognizing that their own product and service output quality depends on quality supplies, components, and raw materials. The increasingly sophisticated purchasing function has learned it can push certain of its costs upstream on supplier-partners. For instance, buying practices waving the "just-in-time" delivery banner often are little more than seller-financed inventory schemes, industrialists have complained.

Intimate information exchange with critically important customers probably will continue to be the best way for manufacturers to innovate in highly complex technical fields. Some companies even invite customers to join new product development teams. And as Professor Eric von Hippel of the Massachusetts Institute of Technology points out in his "lead user" concept, maintaining continuous contact with technically adventuresome customers keeps a company's R&D focus ahead of market trends.

The success of that tack assumes, of course, that a company can adapt its technology fast enough to serve enough of those changing customer requirements. When they cannot and the aforementioned "marketing contradiction" surfaces to spoil the party, the integrators and other intermediaries of the value chain fill the gap. They become the true marketers, linking production to consumption.

The growing power of the channel has proved vexing to marketers in a number of industries through the later 1980s and early 1990s. Ofttimes the distributor and dealer, not the manufacturer, "owns" the customer by earning the loyalty. Although channel power so far has appeared most clearly as a crisis for consumer goods manufacturers, it's a growing peril for manufacturers in business markets, particularly those with weakly differentiated offerings and brand images. Fortunately for them, growing competition among channels provides natural market segmentation, albeit driven by the distributor's strategy rather than the manufacturer's.

Technology's Marketing Face

Technology is also the handmaiden of much-improved marketing practice. The desktop computer revolution of the mid-1980s put marketing people in control of their own data. Concurrent growth in portable computing brought the same benefits to field selling operations. Wired and non-wired communications productivity amplified the power of those tools. Having more control naturally led to more creative use of the data, be it with fine-tuned lead follow-up systems or elaborate expert system and artificial intelligence modeling aids for marketing.

The technologies themselves are tactical-level tools, however. Marketing's challenge is using advanced methods to devise new strategies not otherwise possible. Sales force automation, for instance, must become more than simply speeding up paper and telephone communications. It should enable selling initiatives not otherwise feasible without the technology. Companies that build demonstration and order-configuration tools for salespeople to use with customers find the computer makes the salesperson a more powerful ally of the buyer, a hero to himself and customer alike. In contrast, automation that simply squeezes more speed and productivity out of erstwhile paper reporting systems makes salespeople feel abused by what they see as time-clock efficiency demands.

At corporate headquarters, meanwhile, modern database management abetted by technology should be more than "list maintenance." Systems should constantly analyze and highlight strategic opportunities the firm can exploit. Surviving in fast-action markets of the future will demand it.

Technology can even change the nature of the firm's competitive advantage. Some retail grocery chains have found they made more money from selling their check-out scanner data than from selling the groceries, for example. American Airlines is said to make more from its Sabre computerized airline reservation system than from actually running its airline.

Overcoming Ourselves

Few of these rosy marketing millennium predictions will come true for U.S. marketers unless industry overcomes some persistent cultural obstacles. Most prominent is our pernicious demand for short-term performance gains. In a democracy, the voters get the politicians they deserve. And in a capitalist economy, investors get the long-term thinking they allow, to the extent they allow it at all.

Squeezed by increasing competition and market saturation, business-to-business and consumer-to-business marketers alike have found market growth harder to attain. By the 1990s, simply maintaining market share points no longer reasonably ensured growing revenues. To maintain profit growth, companies cut costs. For many, the incessant short-term pressure of capital markets prompted slash-and-burn attacks on cost centers.

In some cases, of course, bloated organization charts and ill-starred ventures characteristic of the 1980s speculation spirit no longer made sense in the slow-growth 1990s. But for many firms, desperate attempts to shore up P&L statements led to cutting management muscle as well as fat in excessively "downsized" and "flat" organizations. Overworked employees with no time for inspiration will prove to be a major impediment for companies hoping to thrive in 21st-century markets.

The risk-takers benefitting the most from agile marketing strategies are likely to be the smaller, entrepreneurial firms driven by vision rather than cost containment. Their marketing leaders will know how the metrics of their craft translate point-for-point into profit. They will invest enthusiastically in marketing, becoming the vanguard of the business marketing millennium.

–25–
TELEMARKETING

Steven F. Walker

Steven F. Walker is President/CEO of Walker Direct Marketing, L.P., a subsidiary of the Indianapolis based Walker Group of Companies. Walker Group is a 54-year-old management information holding company comprised of six separate entities which together account for over $40 million in sales. Walker has spent the last ten years serving the Walker organization in a variety of capacities, including operations management, account management, sales marketing, analysis, and consulting. He has also published articles and given speeches about marketing research, telemarketing, and database marketing to various industry associations and groups. In 1990, he was instrumental in the founding of Walker Direct as Walker Group's entry into the database marketing industry.

The mention of the word *telemarketing* creates vivid images in the minds of most people and most of these images are not very favorable. Telephone calls at home during dinner from people we do not know, selling us things that we do not need or have no interest in. We picture these people as the modern day equivalent of the snake oil salesman—full-incentive salespeople working in a boiler room environment and being coached to use deceptive and assumptive high-pressure, sales tactics.

To the sophisticated marketer in the year 2000, telemarketing will have an entirely different meaning and image. While the word "telemarketing" has perhaps suffered irreversible damage, the business process and function that it allows will be of increasing importance and value. For purposes of this paper, I would like to introduce the definition that I use for *legitimate telemarketing:* Telemarketing is the planned use of the telephone in traditional and evolving marketing strategies and tactics.

The tremendous growth in popularity of telemarketing is already established. It is the fastest growing advertising medium today, and this growth is projected to continue at rates of over 20 percent annually to the year 2000. By the start of the new century, telemarketing will be an instrumental and valued component of every organization's marketing strategy and every product or service's marketing mix.

Much of the rationalization for why telemarketing has grown has been the rather smug response of "because it works." Closer examination shows that the reasons are much more complex and are consistent with the evolution of marketing in today's fast changing and information-rich marketplace. Examining sophisticated marketers and their evolving applications will confirm this assertion. I would like to examine three specific macro environmental impacts that I believe will cause telemarketing to be even more important by the year 2000.

Telemarketing as a Complement to a Total Quality Management Philosophy

The quality revolution is the future of marketing. It requires that organizations understand their customer's valid requirements on an individual basis. As niche markets become even more specialized, more finite and more defined, we can no longer talk about marketing to clusters. We must talk about servicing each cus-

Futurescope

Telemarketing (and telemarketers) of the future will have shed the reputation for high-pressure, low-quality selling. As organizations develop and use database marketing to understand and service customers better, telemarketing will become an indispensable part of the new marketing environment.

tomer as the individual that he or she is. The tool that is critical to accomplishing this is the database. Tomorrow's marketing database will include all of the pertinent information about an individual customer or prospect and the telephone will be the vehicle of choice to collect and organize this critical data.

With the pace of change increasing at even faster rates, controlling database obsolescence will become a necessity for survival. Organizations that can capture all relevant change going on in the marketplace with both customers and prospects will be the ones most effective at determining customer's requirements and delivering value.

Scrutinization of Marketing Efficiency

The entire premise of direct marketing was first described in the early 1970s. It held that the waste in marketing comes not from reaching those who wish to buy, but from expending resources on those not qualified or not interested in buying. Unlike mass media advertising and traditional sales techniques, telemarketing continues a tradition of direct marketing which directly links consumer behavior to the stimuli applied to the marketplace.

This accountability of effort combined with a systematic approach to eliminating obsolescence will continue to make the telephone an instrumental part of a database marketing environment. The use of the telephone integrated with marketplace databases can directly link advertising with sales and systematically eliminate waste in the sales and marketing processes while quantifying the costs of acquiring and retaining new business.

The Realization of Ethical Telemarketing

Although it may appear to be an oxymoron, "ethical telemarketing" or "the ethical use of the phone in traditional marketing activities" will become the solution to many of the problems currently being raised by privacy advocates and legislative activities. This assertion stems from a basic premise that most customers want their suppliers to know them well and to use their knowledge of their wants and needs to provide better quality products and services at lower and lower costs. The collection of usable marketing information done by honest and trusted suppliers and vendors will create improved customer service and higher customer satisfaction. The ethical problems associated with telemarketing are not created by the technology, but by the values of the people who use the technology.

It is difficult to imagine any business or organization operating without telemarketing applications in the year 2000. We are in an age of information and the ability to organize, retrieve, and utilize information is the key to any success. When integrated into a database marketing strategy, telemarketing, by whatever name it is known, will be the most powerful tool available to accomplish the strategic goals of tomorrow's marketing-driven organization.

Section V
Strategic Marketing Management

The speed of new communications and the general need to make decisions and communicate more quickly create a sense of urgency and immediacy for all functions, yet the need for a strategic vision—of a view of where the marketing organization will be not only tomorrow or next week or next month, but also next year and in the next five years is as crucial to marketing success as it has always been. In "Marketing Strategy: Setting the Course for the New Century," Larry Chiagouris defines the key components of marketing strategy that will drive the company of the future. In "Winning the Marketing Wars," Gerald Michaelson identifies the key lessons to be learned from history's most prominent military strategists. And in "The New Marketing Strategy: Embracing the Future," Ray Lewis explains those lessons in two phrases: creative thinking and solid strategy developed from knowing the customer, knowing how the market is changing, and knowing the environment.

Building and profiting from customer relationships has always been an important element of marketing success. In "Category Management: A Marketing Concept for Changing Times," Doug Adams explores the new uses of marketing information that will enable marketers to manage groups of products to the satisfaction of increasingly fragmented groups of customers. And Terry Vavra and Richard Barlow analyze the strategic dimensions of this issue in "Aftermarketing: The Importance of Retention Marketing" and "Frequency Marketing."

Having a strategic vision is vital to success but so is communicating that vision throughout the organization. In "The Many Views of Integrated Marketing Com-

163

munications," Don Schultz explores the multiple perspectives within and among different types of organizations and explains how they can and must work together to develop effective marketing strategies. In "Marketing Training Beyond 2000," Richard Chvala outlines the steps needed to develop training programs that show the organization's commitment to its mission and that ensure performance at every level. O.C. Ferrell explains the importance of ethics training in marketing in "Ethics Builds Trust in Marketing Relationships." In "Improving Marketing Productivity," Jagdish Sheth and Rajendra Sisodia outline a new approach to marketing productivity—effective efficiency—that responds to the issues and concerns expressed in this section and that, they contend, successful marketers of the future will use to develop more sensible strategies and more effective systems of monitoring and measuring productivity.

–26–
MARKETING STRATEGY
Setting the Course for the New Century

Larry G. Chiagouris

Larry Chiagouris is Executive Vice President, Director of Client and Strategic Services, Creamer Dickson Basford Public Relations and founder of Brand-Marketing Services, Ltd., a strategic marketing and research consulting company. He has served on the board of directors of the American Marketing Association and the Advertising Research Foundation and has counseled many leading packaged goods, services and technology companies, to include AT&T, General Foods, Panasonic, Citibank and Pfizer. He holds a Ph.D. from CUNY in Marketing and a B.S. in Economics from New York University.

The term *marketing strategy* does not have a definition that the majority of marketing professionals would agree to or use. Not only is there an absence of a consensus concerning the definition, but also there is a significant amount of confusion. The definition for purposes of this discussion is grounded in the manner in which a firm manages its resources. Specifically, marketing strategy is the overriding principle a firm uses to organize and allocate its resources to generate profit from customers that are, in the aggregate, part of a market with reasonably clear parameters concerning its size and components. There are several parts to this definition. Each part will serve as a basis for discussing the practical areas of marketing strategy.

First, in terms of the overriding principle that drives a firm's marketing strategy, it is clear that it should be related to the vision that a company has created for its future. This vision should reflect where the firm expects to be positioned in five to ten years. How, in effect, it wants to be perceived. If, for example, a firm desires to be the leader in fashion apparel, then its marketing strategy for an apparel division or brand would reflect this objective. As an overriding principle based on its resource limitations and market analysis, it might establish a marketing strategy that it will serve only leading department stores and cater to fashion-conscious young adults (who tend to set fashion trends). Its market strategy must fit with its vision and this, in turn, will probably vary as its focus becomes more narrow and goes from holding company to division to brand.

What is considered strategy to one individual might be considered tactics to another. A more narrow focus, such as for a brand, will result in strategic direction that appears more tactical. In the end, the marketing strategy will shape the manner in which the firm allocates resources through manipulation of the marketing mix. In addition, organization of its employees with emphasis on marketing, sales, and research and development will also be affected. Vendor selection and raw material acquisition could also be influenced by strategic direction.

The development of a marketing strategy requires fundamental assessment of both the firm and the market. The chosen strategy should be the one that is thought to be best at leveraging a firm's assets in pursuit of the market that it has selected

Futurescope

In order to meet the 21st century on their own terms, companies must establish a comprehensive marketing strategy. The fierce competition of the future will not allow for marketers that have not carefully assessed their marketing operations, brand images, and potential markets. This assessment will guide the firm's vision of its position and prospects in the coming century.

as its focus. Three fundamental tools have been successful in helping guide the process of choosing a strategic direction: the marketing audit, market potential assessment, and brand essence.

The Marketing Audit

An all-inclusive examination of a company's or brand's entire marketing operation as measured against corporate or division growth objectives and industry-wide norms is known as a marketing audit. It is performed by a team consisting of outside marketing specialists and in-house personnel from finance and/or research. Together they map the critical elements as to strengths and weaknesses of the firm, resource constraints, and achievability of current business objectives, all within the context of the current or proposed competitive frame. It is not unusual to find that the firm lacks consensus about any of these elements. The marketing audit is used to arrive at a consensus that will assure an efficient, common sense of purpose.

Market Potential Assessment

Market potential assessment fully documents all critical "need-to-know" aspects of a proposed business (e.g., the state of the category or categories under consideration, financial considerations, trends, prospect analyses, competitive profiles, full advertising analyses, pricing, and other marketing support programs). The final result includes an estimate of the size and components of potential markets that would be appropriate for business development.

Critical to this part of the process is the specification of the source of business that is to be considered the basis for additional revenue. The source of business will ultimately drive many subsequent tactical decisions concerning targeting and marketing mix changes to appeal to the agreed on targets. Although the source of business can be specified in a variety of ways, generally there are three primary sources:

1. Increased revenue (usage) from existing customers

2. Revenue from competitors' customers

3. Revenue from prospects who are not currently category users

The marketing audit provides an examination of the firm. The market potential assessment provides an examination of the potential markets that the firm might enter or further develop. The final step to strategy development prior to implementation of tactics concerns the brand and another key tool, brand essence.

Brand Essence

Brand essence is a layering process that dissects a company-wide (e.g., AT&T, Coke, Avis) or a product-specific brand (e.g., Pampers, PS-2, Advil). The brand is decomposed into its key components: attributes, benefits, values, and personality. At the conclusion of this step, a blueprint for the brand is established that assures all subsequent tactics will reflect the inner core identity of the brand, a process critical to effective strategy execution.

In conclusion, marketing strategy, while an abstract term, ultimately must be applied to provide direction to the firm's business activities. The direction results in a definition of the market to be pursued as well as the profitable allocation of financial resources, human resources, and manipulation of the marketing mix. The result of an effective strategy is the ability to meet the future on favorable terms and sustain financial growth.

—27—
WINNING THE
MARKETING WAR

Gerald A. Michaelson

Gerald A. Michaelson is an experienced corporate executive who has worked for several Fortune 500 companies. He is Executive Vice President of Tennessee Associates International, a management consulting firm based in Knoxville, Tennessee. This article is based on his book *Winning the Marketing War,* which has been acclaimed as the best book on strategy ever written.

In 1925, a Chinese historian was asked to identify the lessons of the French Revolution. "I would love to," he responded, "but it is still too early to tell." Evidence is strong that the relatively short marketing history of less than 50 years is a hodgepodge of information that has yet to congeal. Today's managers can learn more from over 2,000 years of war than they can from 50 years of marketing history.

The Chinese strategist, Sun Tzu, wrote *The Art of War* in 500 B.C. and laid the foundation for Eastern military strategy, which is based on the concept that winning requires good planning. Sun Tzu says that those who are really skilled in battle can subdue the enemy's army without fighting. The German general Carl von Clausewitz, who wrote *On War* in the 18th century, supplies the foundation for Western military strategy, in which the key idea is that to win, one must fight the big battle.

Eastern and Western Military Strategy

Properly understood, Eastern and Western military strategy offer great value to business strategy:

Sun Tzu's thinking is focused on the strategic side of business, doing the right thing, which is marketing.

Clausewitz contributes to the tactical side of business, doing things right, which is selling.

Where does strategy (marketing) end and tactics (selling) begin? Admiral Mahon, in his book on sea power, said, "Contact is a word which perhaps better than any other indicates the dividing line between strategy and tactics." Strategy stops at the border in war. It stops at the headquarters door in business. When the president of the company is talking to a customer, the action is tactical. When the sales manager is planning calls on the customer, the action is strategic.

Futurescope

Taking lessons from strategists writing hundreds or thousands of years ago can be the best preparation for launching marketing attacks in the years to come. In an increasingly complex, global marketplace, marketers cannot afford to overlook the Eastern or the Western philosophies of conquest. A multinational future will be dominated by those who can focus their resources at the most vulnerable areas of the market.

The writings of the great strategists do not tell us exactly how to conduct business strategy or tactics. Rather, they serve as reflectors to help us interpret what we know by providing a means of comparing our own strategies with fundamental strategic concepts.

Marketing Strategy According to Sun Tzu

There are over 100 different translations of Sun Tzu into Japanese and only a handful into English. Sun Tzu can be confusing and frustrating to Western minds, which desire specific systems. *The Art of War* does not offer a system but rather is a series of conceptual statements. Here are examples that can be readily applied to business.

- **"A victorious army seeks its victories before seeking battle, an army destined to defeat fights in the hope of winning."** In business, winning strategies are formulated before the sale. If not, competitive battles take place in the marketplace. I've found that when my strategy was strong enough, I've had little competition. Enviable positions of strength have been occupied by companies like Procter & Gamble in detergents, Microsoft in software, and Wal-Mart in retailing.

- **"Know your enemy and know yourself; and in a hundred battles you will never be defeated."** Information can help achieve victory. When I know the character and personality of my competitors as individuals and as a corporation, I can better predict how they will act in the future. Patterns are repeated. Know what they've done, and you know what they will do.

- **"Use the normal to engage; the extraordinary to win."** Little bits of effort get little bits of results. Too many business plans are little more than an engagement with the competitor and achieve no significant increase in position with the customer. Only when I develop extraordinary plans do I achieve extraordinary success. Anything less is just a dance.

- **"The ultimate strategy is to subdue the enemy's army without engaging it. To take his cities without laying siege to them. To overthrow his forces without blooding swords."** The ultimate sales strategy is to subdue the competitor without having to sell against him. To take his accounts without spending a lot of time. To beat the competition without red ink.

Military Tactics According to Clausewitz

Clausewitz has the most business credibility with managers who are action oriented. His greatest contributions to tactical success can be found in the principles of absolute and relative superiority in *On War:*

- **Absolute superiority.** "The superiority in numbers is the most important factor in the result of a combat, consequently the greatest possible number of troops should be brought into action at the decisive point."

- **Relative superiority.** "Where absolute superiority is not attainable, you must produce a relative one at the decisive point by making skillful use of what you have."

I've won only when I've achieved some kind of absolute or relative superiority. Often we do not have absolute superiority and must find a relative one. The customer will pay your price only if they see a distinct relative superiority in your product or service.

Although relative superiority is most easily thought of as the weight of sheer numbers, it can be achieved in any element of the marketing mix. Success has been achieved with plans designed to achieve relative superiority at the point of contact in training, credit, warranty, service, salesmanship, etc.

Efforts where not enough resources are concentrated at the decisive place and time result in all of the resources being wasted. The decision concerning how many resources to concentrate is related to what it takes and what the competitor is doing. Whenever I've tried to replace a competitor, I've had to concentrate enough strength to dislodge that competitor. Being as good as the competitor wasn't good enough. That didn't cause change. The product or service had to be considerably better.

The way to win is to plan "win win." Plan a winning strategy that will beat the competition and excite the customer. Plan winning tactics for delivering that strategy to the customer.

The Principles of the Marketing War

A principle is a guide that can never be ignored. Following the principles does not guarantee that you will win. Ignore the principles and you will surely lose. A review of a few of the key principles yields insight into how to convert them to practical business applications:

Developing the Plan
Organization of intelligence:
Know your market as well as you know yourself.
The objective:
Have a clear intention and steady aim.
A secure position:
Occupy a position that cannot easily be taken by your opponents.

Launching the Attack
Offensive action:
Keep on the offensive to assure freedom of action.

Surprise:
The best way to gain psychological dominance and deny the initiative to your opponent is the art of surprise.
Maneuver:
The easiest routes are the most heavily defended; the longest way 'round can be the shortest way home.
Concentration of resources:
Mass sufficiently superior force at the decisive place and time.

Managing the Battle

Economy of force:
Assess accurately where you employ your resources.
Command structure:
The management process unleashes the power of human resources.
Personal leadership:
Success requires the leader's faith in his people, and their faith in his ability to win.
Simplicity:
Even the simplest plans are difficult to execute.

Organization of Intelligence

Intelligence has always been vital to the success of military operations. Every command has its own intelligence section. Business intelligence systems focus on both the competitor and the customer. The business battleground is the customer's mind. In a real sense, it is a mental struggle in which you try to outthink your competitors. To achieve success in this mental struggle, accurate information is essential.

Concentration of Resources

The principle of concentration of resources is one of the primary principles of war used by armies throughout the world. Clausewitz says, "Concentrate sufficiently superior resources at the decisive place and time." B.H. Liddell Hart says, "You must have as much as you can for yourself and as little for the enemy." Sun Tzu says:

When ten to the enemy's one, surround him.
When five times his strength, attack him.
If double his strength, divide him.
If equally matched, you may engage him.
If weaker numerically, be capable of withdrawing.

And if in all respects unequal, be capable of eluding him, for a small force is but booty for one more powerful.

We win where we concentrate forces. Time after time, the big guys win. However, the concentration does not have to be of overall superiority. We can win by having superiority in a segment, or in a small segment called a niche.

Maneuver

The most common maneuver is the flanking attack. MacArthur did it at Inchon. Schwarzkopf did it in the war with Iraq. Clausewitz says, "Flank and rear attacks are by far the most successful." The essence of a business flanking is the end run around the competitor's position to a lightly defended position in the market. Procter & Gamble flanked with Crest. Land did it with a camera. Wal-Mart's initial location strategy was to flank other mass merchants by going to small towns.

Military strategy and tactics are not a good source for business strategy and tactics, they are a great choice. The great generals should not be regarded as seminal sources of specific information, but rather as a way to help shape and simplify one's own thinking.

—28—
THE NEW
MARKETING
STRATEGY
Embracing the Future

J. Raymond Lewis, Jr.

J. Raymond Lewis, Jr. joined Holiday Inn Worldwide in 1985, after nearly two decades of experience in sales, marketing, and advertising. He is currently Executive Vice President of Worldwide Sales & Marketing. Lewis is a member of the board and executive committee of Holiday Inn Worldwide, and is a member of the Association of National Advertisers and the National Advertising Review Board. He has also served on the Services Marketing Council of the American Marketing Association and is a member of the American Management Association. In addition, he has been active in a number of civic organizations.

The greatest threat to an organization's marketing success today is blind acceptance of fantasies, whether they're truly outrageous ideas or just everyday fantasies. Fantasies are any type of theory or opinion that's based on looking backwards.

There can be no future success for anyone—individuals or companies—that operate according to "because I said so" or "that's the way it is." There will be no success for those who follow the "that's the way we've always done it" mentality, no success for any group that chooses to believe that today is like yesterday, ignoring the implications of the clear-cut revolution that's affecting every aspect of business today.

If we began to list the changes in our society just over the last 5 or 10 years—things like changing consumer lifestyles, distribution systems, value orientation, globalization, world economy—there would be almost nothing untouched. For each of those changes, there must be a new set of rules.

But, being products of our environment, we follow Newton's law. We're objects in motion, and we continue along the same path until something with sufficient force stops us. And it usually takes something like a brick wall.

Blind acceptance of the status quo leads us to do things like look at the economy and say, "Well, it looks sort of like a recession. It sounds like a recession. It must be a recession." Then we react like we always have. We go into the old traditional bunker mentality: cut costs, tighten our belts, and clench our teeth till it passes. It worked in the past. But it won't work today. Because we're not in a typical recession. Recession is far too simplistic a term for the complete economic restructuring we're experiencing. The last few years should have been our economic brick wall.

The Changing Marketing Environment

It's not just the financial climate that's at issue here. The geopolitical realities that have been spawned by the fall of the Berlin Wall and subsequent revolutionary changes have created a new environment, an environment that's not a temporary situation, like a recession. It's a permanent social, political, and economic change. And all of those factors dramatically affect the way consumers think, feel, and act.

What that means for successful marketers is that we're moving swiftly into a twilight zone of business trends. An uncharted galaxy of consumer implications.

We've moved through the age of financial manipulation—that was the 1980s. We've entered the age of marketing—that's the 1990s and beyond. And it's a dimension of marketing where no man . . . or woman . . . has gone before, where understanding the consumer—and the changing needs of that consumer—is every bit as important as understanding financial maneuvers or utilizing technology.

There is no more boom town: create a product and then wait for people to line up to buy it. Competition is stiff and getting stiffer. Look at the industrialized

---

Futurescope

The old formulas for success are dead. Marketing success in the future will be determined by a combination of creative thinking and solid strategy that comes from knowing what the customer wants, continuously measuring and responding to changes in the market, and recognizing the demands of the new global environment.

---

world. Many markets have reached maturity. And in such markets, the only way we can be successful is to create our own economic advantage by stealing share.

The only companies that will be successful in the 1990s and beyond are the ones that use their marketing ingenuity to learn how to steal market share. They'll have to forget everything they used to know and look at things through a new pair of glasses. Through those glasses they'll clearly identify *changing* consumer needs, and then they'll use all their power to meet those needs. In this day, clever marketing is the only way to increase competitive edge in the marketplace.

Marketing doesn't mean a bundle of programs and promotions. That's the old definition of marketing. Marketing is not only a department. It's no longer a separate discipline or an add-on to corporate strategy. Marketing *is* the strategy.

Success in the 1990s will depend upon our ability to think innovatively not just about our business environment, but also about the entire marketing process. Strong competitors will look at things differently, and then have the courage to stand up and make things change.

An examination of the *Fortune* 500 list reveals that past success is not necessarily a predictor of future success, that just because things have always been one way does not guarantee that they'll be that way forever. Many companies have dropped off the list in recent years. Some sources cite adherence to hierarchical thinking as a major contributor to the employment declines that have occurred every year since 1980 (with the exception of 1985, a flat year).

Increases in employment and profitability have come from the 4 or 5 percent of the fastest growing companies dedicated to identifying well-defined consumer needs and rapidly and excellently satisfying those needs. They're the ones taking advantage of the significant growth opportunities in the U.S. GDP. And it's no coincidence that they're radical thinkers, the ones who've taken a creative approach to marketing.

What we're seeing is a marketing revolution, and today's business leaders are at the forefront of that change.

Look who's on the list today: McDonald's, a company that's kept a very close eye on what consumers want. It's no accident that today you find salads and yogurt and healthier choices on their menus. Home Depot. Office Depot. AST. These companies understand consumer needs and take action to meet them. They ignore what worked in the past because they don't live or operate in the past. They operate in the 1990s. And they do it successfully.

Intel is one of my favorite stories. In the 1980s everyone gave Intel up for dead, along with the U.S. microchip market. Then what happened? Intel developed the 386, and the 486, and then, while they were in court over a patent violation regarding the 486, they were busy inventing a whole new technology: the Pentium chip. They planned their own obsolescence.

These are examples of the kind of innovative marketing that will be necessary for the '90s and beyond—not marketing as programs and promotions, but marketing as strategy, marketing that drives the corporate plan in a very methodical way.

The Steps to Marketing Success

Successful companies didn't just stumble over good ideas. And they certainly didn't wait around for a Fairy Godmother to zap them. They followed a simple formula, doing the things that I define as the 10-step marketing process. Here's what I see innovative companies doing.

1. Understanding the needs of the consumer—doing the research to find out what products and services people want.

2. Understanding what it's going to take to succeed—determining how much of the market share you have to have, how many dollars must you make, and brutally controlling costs to keep them in line with profits. That means smart budgeting that keeps costs in line but never, never scrimps on the user side.

3. Continuously getting feedback and measuring success, not just in terms of how they're doing, but also in terms of how they're doing compared with their competitors.

4. Thinking nontraditionally. Federal Express, for example, defined a whole new market with its overnight deliveries. Mercedes stopped selling cars and started selling social acceptance. Coca-Cola never sold bubbly colored water but always sold refreshment. And as time went on, when refreshment came to mean things like with and without color, with and without caffeine, with and without calories, they were ready to provide them all—because that's what the customer wanted.

5. Defining markets and identifying long-term opportunities in those markets. Simplistically, that means, for instance, figuring out not just what baby boomers want or need today, but what baby boomers will want in 10 or 20 years.

6. Understanding that good value doesn't mean a cheap product. The value equation has two sides. It doesn't only mean what you pay. It means what you *get* for what you pay. In the hotel industry, for example, look at the difference in the success of economy brands. Some companies defined the economy product as a cheap hotel room, and they created a cheap product. A few smart companies, like Red Roof Inn and Hampton Inns, recognized that customers didn't want a cheap room; they wanted a good product at a low price.

   What's required is a solid pricing strategy that's based on market needs, not on how much money you want to make. A strategy that's driven by the value equation: What you pay for what you get.

7. Recognizing the competitive framework. Who is the competition? And what's the best competitive edge? The toughest companies distinguish themselves with things other than bricks and mortar. Competitors can copy tangible things, but they can't copy an operating philosophy and a commitment to excellence.

8. Recognizing the global environment. We're no longer talking about an American market, or a Japanese product, or a German competitor. In the 1950s and 1960s, American auto companies were competing with each other. In the '70s and '80s, they were competing with the Japanese, the Germans, the French, etc. Today, we're forming alliances to create cross-cultural products—expanding to international markets, becoming global companies.

   Companies that limit their ability to compete by drawing geographic boundaries aren't just limiting their success, they're signing their death warrants. How many people take it for granted that American products can't compete with Japanese products? Well, interestingly enough, the most successful maker of cellular phones in Japan is none other than Motorola. Who's making major share gains selling four-wheel-drive vehicles in Japan? Jeep. Contrast that with a few years ago, when American auto manufacturers couldn't make significant headway in Japan. Why? Not necessarily just because of poor American engineering, but because we tried to sell cars with the steering wheel on the left—and all the Japanese toll-booths are on the right. Not poor engineering or manufacturing; inadequate flexibility in understanding and meeting marketing needs.

9. Targeting efforts and prioritizing resources toward those efforts. No one has the luxury of unlimited resources. Resources are finite, and they're too valuable to waste. So, good strategy requires accurate deployment of dollars and people to get the most from the least.

10. Realizing that you can't do everything all the time. The way to win is to focus on a few things and then stay committed to doing them in an outstanding way time after time.

We're in a war for share, and the companies that will win the war don't live according to the old hierarchical belief system. And they don't follow other people's lead. Successful companies today live in the present. They think for themselves. They have a clear picture of today, and they keep a close eye on tomorrow.

The Necessity for New Thinking

Without a fresh mindset, we're destined to live out the story of the proverbial lemmings. Every four years, the little lemmings prance up to the shoreline, dip their toes in and say, "Hmm, the water's fine." And then they all jump in and drown. So what does that tell us? It tells us that the only lemmings that have a fifth birthday party are the ones who think for themselves.

The reality is, there is no fairy godmother to tell us what to do. It's a time for creative thinking, and planning and acting, not in the interest of creating a defensive stand, but in the interest of developing the most aggressive offense we can muster. We must create growth by stealing share from the competition.

Creative thinking. Good strategy. A simple definition of what marketing's all about.

—29—
CATEGORY MANAGEMENT
A Marketing Concept for Changing Times

Doug Adams

Doug Adams is president of the Efficient Consumer Response (ECR) and Operational Applications Division of Nielsen Marketing Research NA. As such, he is responsible for developing and directing the company's ECR activities, including designing and implementing strategies and tactics, products and services, and marketing. He is also responsible for several specific product areas, including coordinating daily store-level data acquisition and processing, ECR software applications, and logistic management systems. Adams has been a regular speaker at industry conferences in the United States and Europe. He holds a bachelor's degree in economics and an M.B.A. in finance and marketing from Emory University.

The fragmentation of the consumer packaged-goods marketplace and the growing use of information technology have created an increasingly complex playing field for retailers and manufacturers competing for market share in the 1990s. These same factors also have led to the growing use of an innovative new marketing concept known as *category management*.

Rooted in the belief that today's new-product explosion has made strategic management by item impractical and strategic management by department unfocused, category management is a process that involves managing product categories as business units and customizing each category's product mix, merchandising, and promotions to satisfy customer needs on a store-by-store basis.

Although category management produces merchandising programs tailored to the "little picture" at individual stores, its ultimate goal is to unite these snapshots into a "big picture" that supports a company's mission, image, and strategic objectives.

A Long-Term Process

It's important to remember that category management is a circular, long-term process, not a linear, short-term project. It requires continual evaluation of sales and demographic data to determine who buys what in a particular category, where they buy it, how often, and how much they spend. Information, technology, and applications can help to answer these questions and many others.

Working together, retailers and manufacturers can identify brand-loyal consumers and high-volume shoppers, pinpoint their media preferences, and gauge their responsiveness to specific promotions. They also can determine how the performance of one category affects other categories in the same store.

Futurescope

The lifeblood of category management is market intelligence. It stems from technological advances, including electronic checkout scanners, decision support systems, powerful mainframe applications, and demographic databases. Software applications can then produce information for analyzing pricing, promotions, and shelf space. This information yields market knowledge, which in turn leads to strategies, tactics, and action. Twenty years ago, just having the type of market intelligence that now is widely available would have given any manufacturer or retailer a major competitive advantage. Today, it's not having the information that matters. It's how it's used. And a growing number of manufacturers and retailers are recognizing that they can use it most effectively by implementing category management and then working together to maximize its benefits.

Armed with this data, retailers and manufacturers can develop customized strategies for individual categories in specific stores, based on a retailer's image, a category's strategic role, and a store's location and customer demographics. Specifically, they can tailor category assortments, self-space allocations, pricing, and consumer and trade promotions to maximize sales and profits. Best of all, they can test such strategies before implementing them by using sophisticated computer modeling programs.

Stages of Category Management

Category management involves five ongoing stages, each of which flows naturally into the next, allowing retailers and manufacturers to adapt quickly to marketplace changes. The stages include the following:

1. Reviewing categories

2. Targeting consumers

3. Planning merchandising

4. Implementing strategy

5. Evaluating results

Although the general concepts behind each stage are the same for retailers and manufacturers, there are significant differences in execution and logistics. The process presents numerous opportunities for retailers and manufacturers to help each other to implement the strategy successfully. It's possible to practice category management without such interaction, but the process works best when retailers and manufacturers share their powerful marketing capabilities.

Before implementing category management, retailers and manufacturers must define their mission/image and develop marketing strategies and objectives to further it. In doing so, they must determine what role individual product categories will be expected to play in their corporate game plan, beginning with a clear definition of each category.

This isn't as easy as it might sound, because retailers and market research companies sometimes view a category differently than do manufacturers, and shoppers sometimes have yet another definition.

When in doubt, it's best to err on the side of the consumer, especially in a category that has any products that, from a consumer point of view, could be substituted for each other. Third-party data can help retailers and manufacturers get a handle on consumer perceptions of a category. A good rule of thumb is that products that are substituted for each other should be grouped in the same category.

As the definition of each category comes into focus, retailers and manufacturers must make sure to identify important subcategories that can significantly influence the performance of the category as a whole. It's important to understand the trends that drive each subcategory and to determine the impact the subcategory has on other products—in the same category and across categories.

Similarly, retailers and manufacturers should understand how one category's performance can affect another's. For example, the fortunes of the beverage and snacks categories often are intertwined.

At this stage, retailers also must align individual categories with their corporate mission/image and overall marketing and financial objectives. What strategic role is each category best suited to play? Is it an image enhancer? A traffic or sales builder? A profit builder?

Third-party research data can be used to assess the category's position in a retailer's stores versus the marketplace as a whole and to answer questions such as: How do I fare by category against my competitors? What is my volume? What is my market share? What are my short-term and long-term growth possibilities? Once these questions have been answered, the retailer can decide how much capital to invest in each category and can establish sales, profit, and market-share objectives for each category.

Building Strategic Alliances

In addition to defining categories, retailers and manufacturers must begin to look at themselves, and each other, in a much different way in order to implement category management successfully.

They must redesign their organizations, integrating merchandising functions with buying or selling responsibilities. Category management involves transforming retail "buyers" and manufacturer "sellers" into entrepreneurs, each responsible for a small business within a larger enterprise.

Within manufacturing companies, this process is fostering the development of a team approach to selling that breaks down communications barriers among sales, marketing, research, and MIS departments and is leading to enhanced operational efficiencies. Similarly, category management is leading retailers to integrate the purchasing function with sales and merchandising.

Retailers and manufacturers also must push aside adversarial feelings to develop mutually beneficial strategic alliances based on sharing market intelligence. To a large extent, market forces already are pushing retailers and manufacturers in this direction.

Faced with a proliferation of retail store formats and a blurring of the lines between trade channels, retailers are searching for new ways to attract and retain savvy customers, and manufacturers are looking for new ways to reach market niches with their product messages and to sell savvy retailers on their brands. The manufacturer is concerned primarily with building brand equity; the retailer wants to build an image as a company that meets specific consumer needs.

Both parties are recognizing the need to work together to fully capitalize on the potential of information, technology, and applications. Both parties, of course, want to increase volume and profitability.

Category management provides a common framework to support the development of long-term, mutually beneficial relationships. By working together on category management, each party can help the other achieve its goals.

Retailers, for example, might have access to more market information than ever, but they often don't have the time to analyze it thoroughly to identify significant consumer and category trends. Many still rely on manufacturers for expertise and guidance in this regard. It's common for retailers to appoint a leading manufacturer as the "captain" for a particular category and then to rely on that manufacturer for category insights and strategic recommendations that can boost volume and profitability.

Manufacturers, on the other hand, might have extensive information about brand performance, but they might not be aware of certain nuances of consumer behavior or competitive activity at individual stores. Retailers can help them fill in these blanks by sharing local-market intelligence.

Reviewing the Category

After defining categories, redefining job functions and relationships, and initiating strategic alliances, retailers and manufacturers can proceed to work together on the five stages of category management.

The first stage, reviewing the category, requires the gathering and integration of a broad range of internal and external data about a specific category.

Essential pieces of information for the manufacturer include the category's unit and dollar volume and growth rates, both on a national basis and by retail trade channel, the level of advertising and promotional activity within the category, and the number of new products introduced into the category during the last year.

The manufacturer also should examine national household purchasing patterns, including how many households buy products from the category, where they shop, and how much they spend. Manufacturers should also chart the performance of its brands versus those of competitors at the national, market, and retail-account levels. This will enable the manufacturer to identify growth opportunities and to capitalize on them by developing new or modified marketing strategies.

The retailer, meanwhile, must analyze and compare the historical performance of a category in the retailer's stores versus the marketplace as a whole, answering questions such as:

• What is our market share in this category?

• What products are hot? Which aren't?

• Which subcategories are trending up? Which are trending down?

- How are consumer and trade promotions affecting the performance of specific products and the category as a whole?

- How does the category's product mix, pricing, shelf-space allocations, promotions, and location within the store compare with competitors'?

Targeting Consumers

During the next stage of category management, targeting consumers, the retailer and manufacturer must identify target customers for a particular category and must strive to understand their lifestyles, shopping habits, media preferences, and needs.

For the manufacturer, this stage involves building a demographic profile of the typical buyer, both for the category and for a specific brand; analyzing general information about the lifestyles of target consumers; and planning promotion and media strategies based on the media preferences of target consumers.

By matching the consumer profile of a brand to a profile of consumers within the trade areas of individual stores, a manufacturer can determine not only a brand's potential within a specific store, but also the potential for a brand's buyers to improve category performance at a particular site. The manufacturer also can determine the most effective product mix, pricing, promotion, and merchandising for doing so.

The retail category manager, meanwhile, focuses on identifying "clusters," or groups of consumers with similar demographic and psychographic characteristics, and then grouping stores whose trading areas include similar clusters. Once the category manager has grouped the stores, he or she can use market research to understand the shopping behavior of the clusters that characterize each group.

Computer software programs are available that can integrate market research with a retailer's own scanning data to help the category manager answer countless questions about the purchase behavior of specific clusters. The answers to these questions allow the category manager to zero in on target customers—those who account for the greatest percentage of sales in the category—and to tailor the product mix, pricing, shelf-space allocations, merchandising, and promotions to meet these customers' needs and to increase store traffic.

Planning Merchandising

The third stage of category management, planning merchandising, involves developing a detailed strategy for product mix, pricing, promotion, and shelf-space allocation within a category. The manufacturer develops customized strategies by retail account; the retailer works with the manufacturer to develop customized strategies for store clusters.

Both parties can use software applications to do the following:

- Determine for which of the manufacturer's brands a particular retailer does not have strong volume potential for both parties.

- Recommend an optimum product mix by projecting the volume and profit gains a retailer would realize by adding such items to its product mix and removing other items.

- Model the effect of different pricing strategies on gross margins for an entire store, a department, a category, or individual items.

- Test different promotion scenarios from the retailer's perspective and the manufacturer's perspective to develop a mutually beneficial strategy. Key variables, such as free standing inserts, seasonality, holidays, deal terms and allowances, forward buying, and shelf space, can be built into models to show how a promotion might affect the performance of a particular brand and the category as a whole.

- Produce planograms showing the most appropriate and profitable product mix and shelf-space allocations for a category in specific types of stores.

- Issue inventory replenishment schedules for like items within a planogram so a manufacturer can better time its shipments to a retailer—a "must" in an environment in which retailers are relying increasingly on just-in-time delivery.

Implementing Strategy

The first major test for any category marketing and merchandising strategy comes during the fourth stage of category management, implementing strategy. At this point, the manufacturer's team sales leader makes a presentation to the category buyer at the retail account for which the strategy was devised. Using information gleaned during the first three steps of the category management process, the team sales leader provides an overview of the category, brands, and consumer purchasing patterns.

The team sales leader then delivers recommendations about product mix, pricing, promotions, and shelf-space strategies, supporting his or her case with charts, tables, planograms, and other output from analyses conducted while planning merchandising for the category. He or she also relates these recommendations to the demographics of the retailer's target customers and to the retailer's financial objectives, explaining how the proposed strategies will help the retailer attract more customers to its stores and improve category volume and profits. Implementing strategy isn't confined to one presentation to a retail buyer. It's a long process that requires a continuing dialogue between the manufacturer and the retailer.

Once a retailer finalizes a strategy for a particular category, the retail category manager and specialists communicate the specifics of their pricing, merchandising, and promotional tactics to store managers, who disseminate instructions to store employees. They then perform the hands-on work involved with pricing changes, product sorting, display assembling and positioning, and other tasks.

Evaluating Results

The fifth stage of category management, evaluating results, is as critical to the process as pedals are to a bicycle. That's because it involves questions, answers, and decisions that keep the circular process flowing naturally back into its first stage, reviewing the category.

The basic question to be answered is: "Did my strategies achieve their objectives?" Today's sophisticated software applications can help manufacturers and retailers answer this question and many others. These applications convert scanning statistics and other market data into actionable knowledge. And they allow manufacturers and retailers to do this faster than ever. Automated computer systems, in fact, can be programmed to digest large amounts of market data and produce on a regular schedule customized reports on the performance of brands and categories.

This knowledge can help retailers' category managers and manufacturers' sales and brand managers to identify new opportunities and unforseen challenges in the marketplace. They then must decide if and how to modify their strategies. These decisions require managers to review their category once again, providing the link that makes category management a dynamic, ongoing process.

Everyone Benefits

Manufacturers and retailers who develop strategic alliances within the framework of category management can realize multiple benefits. Building close relationships with retailers, for example, can enhance a manufacturer's ability to target merchandising and promotions to individual stores.

In essence, category management permits manufacturers to be more efficient at marketing and working with the retailer. Through category management, manufacturers can bring an expanded knowledge base to retailers that benefits both parties. This enables manufacturers to display their commitment to their retail customers' success. For both manufacturers and retailers, category management heightens awareness of consumer needs and brings a consumer-oriented focus to business strategies.

The process allows retailers to "micro-merchandise" by managing their business based on the way people shop it. The retailer who practices category management uses consumer preferences as a guide when dealing with important issues such as:

- What items to carry, in
- What quantity, at
- What prices, in
- What stores, with
- What shelf space, with
- What promotions, at
- What locations in the store, for
- What period of time

At the same time, category management improves asset management by enabling retailers to manage product mix, shelf space, inventory, and capital more effectively. It helps them to maximize their return on their information-technology investment by providing a framework for integrating and interpreting the abundant sales and demographic data now available.

Category management also improves retailers' and manufacturers' ability to assess the impact of advertising and promotions and to modify them as necessary. It allows them to respond quickly to unexpected changes in the marketplace, whether they affect an entire category at several stores or a specific brand within a certain category at a single store, as well as to avoid out-of-stocks. Through category management, retailers and manufacturers can also identify and capitalize on cross-merchandising and cross-promotional opportunities between categories, such as beverages and snack foods.

The strategic alliances spawned by category management improve the retailer's ability to build its image and to offer customized product assortments, merchandising, and promotions. They also enhance the manufacturer's ability to build brand image and equity and bolster both parties' ability to respond effectively to customer needs.

Retailers and manufacturers who understand and share a commitment to category management, strategic alliances, and the tools of information, technology, and applications can provide customers with the products they want, when they want them, at competitive prices. By doing so, they can maximize their profits in today's highly competitive consumer products marketplace.

—30—

THE MANY VIEWS OF INTEGRATED MARKETING COMMUNICATIONS

Don E. Schultz

Don E. Schultz, Ph.D., is a professor of Integrated Marketing Communications at the Medill School of Journalism at Northwestern University. In 1974, he gave up his position as Senior Vice President of Tracy-Locke Advertising and Public Relations to launch his career in academia. He obtained his master's degree in advertising and his Ph.D. in mass media from Michigan State University, and joined Northwestern in 1977. Schultz has written, consulted, held seminars, and lectured extensively on sales, marketing, advertising, and integrated marketing communications, is active in numerous professional organizations, and is President of Agora, Inc., a marketing, advertising, and consulting firm.

Integrated marketing communications (IMC) is an elusive concept. It has as many definitions as it has founders, all of which are legitimate, for IMC is a concept that means many different things to many different people. It all depends on what you are trying to do with the concept and your purpose in doing so. In this brief review, four approaches to or definitions of IMC are discussed. They are from the view of (1) the marketer, (2) the marketing communications agency (advertising, sales promotion, public relations, direct marketing), (3) the media, and (4) the academic or strategic business theory builder.

How the Marketing Organization Views Integrated Marketing Communications

In its most basic form, and from the point of view of the marketing organization, IMC is an attempt to coordinate and consolidate all the marketing communications programs for a company, a brand, or a product line. The primary belief of most marketing executives is that all promotional activities and communictions support for the brand should reflect a consistent image or message or feeling for what is being promoted. Therefore, terminology such as "one sight–one sound," "seamless communications," or "consistent imagery which reflects the essence of the brand" are used to describe their activities. The marketing belief, which stems from the mass production/mass marketing/mass media approaches of the 1960s and 1970s, is that consistency in message look, feel, content, and image are needed and provide a more powerful selling approach than multiple concepts or images or messages.

Although it would seem to be simple for marketing organizations to integrate their communications programs, the development of functional specialists such as advertising managers, sales promotion experts, and direct marketing groups within the corporate structure make this a most difficult task. Thus, for the marketing orga-

Futurescope

Marketing communications planners of the 21st century, faced with proliferation of media outlets and fragmentation of consumer markets, must take integration beyond the "consistent image" approach. This will entail strategic use of consumer purchase data to plan marketing messages based on individual or household behavior. The successful marketer of the future will focus on long-term relationships with customers, rather than on one transaction at a time.

nization, IMC is an attempt to create some order from the multiple voices that the brand and the organization often present to customers and prospects.

The Agency's View of Integrated Marketing Communications

From the view of the agency, IMC is somewhat different. Traditionally, advertising agencies created or helped create most of the marketing communications programs for their clients' products or services. During the 1970s, as national advertising became the most important element in many manufacturers' brand communication efforts, advertising agencies moved away from the so-called support or "below-the-line" functions of sales promotion, packaging, direct marketing, and the like. New, specialized agencies developed in these areas to serve the needs of the functional specialists who were also developing at the same time in the client organizations.

As the retail trade consolidated and concentrated in the late 1970s and early 1980s, more of the brand marketing and communication funds began to be invested in the support areas of trade promotion, direct marketing, consumer promotion, and the like. Because advertising agencies saw their traditional media billings decline as client funds were shifted to these other areas, they began to acquire representatives in the specialized agency field. The belief was that if the client wanted public relations assistance, the advertising agency would offer it.

Thus, from the advertising agency's view, integration of the marketing communications programs was an attempt to retain client billings and to cross-sell the services of the agencies they had acquired. IMC therefore means something totally different to the advertising agencies. Today, as all types of agencies attempt to provide greater service and therefore generate greater income from clients, IMC now often means the integration of various functional agencies or activities to provide a common core of service to clients. To many agencies, IMC is primarily providing a range of services regardless of whether communications programs themselves are integrated in form and function.

How the Media View Ingetrated Marketing Communications

The media view of IMC is similar to that of the agency. Many media organizations have moved from being single-media groups, such as a common ownership and management of several television stations or magazines, to multimedia giants such as Time-Warner, Gannett, Meredith Publishing, Turner Broadcasting, and Viacom. As these media organizations grew and either acquired or invented new forms of media, the natural inclination was to try to find some way to bring them all together under a common selling banner. IMC has provided a viable approach.

Using an IMC approach, Time-Warner or Meredith can offer joint advertising and promotional programs, not just for their various individual media forms such as magazines, but they can also combine media forms as well, such as over-the-air broadcast, cable, and special publications. Indeed, some of these media organizations are busy building or developing other ancillary areas such as customer and consumer databases that will assist them in better integrating all of their media forms to provide greater services to the marketer or advertiser. So, from the media view, IMC is a tool by which multimedia organizations can coordinate and cooperatively offer potential advertisers their entire range of media and promotional alternatives.

Integrated Marketing Communications from the View of the Strategist or Theory Builder

From the view of the business strategist or academic theory builder, IMC is a new concept and process and perhaps even a new theory of how to understand consumers and therefore to build more effective and efficient marketing communications programs.

Traditionally, marketers, their agencies, and the media have looked at and developed marketing communications programs using an "inside-out" approach based on the concept of a hierarchy of effects communication model. Using this mass communication theory, these marketers first developed the goals for the marketing communications programs. Then they developed the communications messages and, finally, selected the media vehicles to deliver those messages to a previously defined (often by demographics only) audience.

The idea of the hierarchy of effects model was that consumers moved through a linear, step-by-step process on the way to a purchase. Generally that movement was based on attitudinal changes. A common version of the process was that the purchase cycle consisted of the customer moving from awareness to knowlege to preference to conviction to purchase. Thus, communications programs were planned to move consumers along that linear path toward purchase. This approach, which is still the basis for most marketing communications programs, assumes that with enough favorable messages, the consumer can be moved to purchase. In other words, the marketing organization develops messages, delivers them to the consumer, and the consumer moves toward purchase.

With the availability of consumer purchase data, instead of a hierarchy of effects approach, the IMC planner looks first at consumer behavior from the "outside-in." In other words, the IMC communications planner looks initially at what consumers have done. He or she then tries to explain that behavior and to reconstruct the concepts, messages, and approaches that led to this behavior.

In reversing the approach, the IMC planner is much more oriented toward individual or household behavior than mass market behavior, and is more interested in behavior than in attempts at prediction. The IMC approach being developed by these strategists and academics looks more at long-term relations with the consumer than does the traditional transaction-oriented marketing communications programs presently in use. Finally, the IMC approach views the actual communications tactics as being derived from consumer and customer behavior and analysis rather than from investment weight or message delivery efficiencies, which have been the basis for most marketing communications programs since the development of mass media.

What is integrated marketing communications? Today, it depends on your view of the marketplace and your marketing communications objectives. IMC is a creature of many shapes and sizes and quite truly is defined primarily in the eyes of the beholder.

—31—
AFTERMARKETING
The Importance of
Retention Marketing

Terry G. Vavra

Terry Vavra is Associate Professor of Marketing at the Lubin School of Business at Pace University in New York. Dr. Vavra is a specialist in customer retention strategies, and is author of the book *Aftermarketing: How to Keep Customers for Life through Relationship Marketing.* In addition to his teaching, he also serves as the president of Marketing Metrics, Inc., a consulting and customer retention firm located in Paramus, New Jersey. His clients include Cellular One, Dentsu Inc., Ferrari, IBM, Motorola, Rolls-Royce, and Seiko Instruments. Dr. Vavra is regularly sought as a speaker for international seminars, and has spoken on American marketing techniques to Canadian, French, Japanese, South American, and British audiences.

U.S. marketing has for too long chased new customers in sometimes futile efforts to increase market share. When the focus has been on conquest marketing, current customers have often received the short end of the stick. Marketers spend hundreds of millions of dollars attempting to win new customers, while evidencing little care or concern for those customers already buying their products and services. Consequently, current customers often defect to other marketers in search of more personalized attention, making it necessary for the marketer to attract new customers.

At one time, the U.S. marketplace was expanding so robustly that efforts to attract new customers were often successful. However, today's marketplace is dramatically different. New customers are harder to find and to attract. Consider the plateauing of population, GNP, and household incomes and the oversaturation of categories with parity brands.

Keeping customers also makes economic sense. Lost customers mean lost revenue: not only the revenue they generated directly, but the opportunity revenue from other potential customers they will dissuade from buying from the organization. Then there are the marketing costs required to win additional customers to replace the lost customers. Costs of losing customers snowball significantly from the seemingly small loss of one customer's account.

But if customers are retained, the longer they stay as customers the more they will depend on a company's products or services, and the less susceptible they will be to other companies' offers. Consequently, a customer's lifetime value can increase dramatically as his or her lifetime with a marketer is extended.

The observation that too many marketers are still singlemindedly pursuing conquest marketing is borne out in a survey conducted among marketing and advertising directors of the country's 100 largest advertisers. These corporate marketing directors confirmed that advertising (primarily a conquest tool) receives 75 percent of their budgets, with only 25 going to all other marketing tools—only some of which are customer retention activities. In contrast, data shows that two-thirds of a business's income comes from current customers.

Futurescope

In the 21st century, smart marketers will focus on strategies designed to retain current customers by increasing their satisfaction, by bonding them to brands and to marketing organizations. The customer-conquest marketing techniques of yesterday are no longer effective. U.S. marketers need to develop retention marketing strategies to survive in the radically different market of tomorrow.

Creating customers requires one set of actions and strategies, a conquest outlook; retaining customers requires a quite different perspective, a retention outlook. And the view of the company-customer relationship as ongoing runs directly against the mindset of a sales-driven company. In sales-driven companies, a sale is considered as *culminating* the contact with customers. But from buyers' perspectives, a sale is likely to be viewed as *initiating* a relationship—the buyer desiring or anticipating continued interaction with the selling company.

Aftermarketing is how to build and strengthen these critically important customer relationships. Aftermarketing encompasses the whole range of activities that a marketer can engage in after a customer has committed to the marketer's brand, product, or service. Although some areas of marketing (database and direct marketing) appear extraordinarily attuned to the value of customer retention, many marketers are not yet switched on. Mainstream marketers must recognize that the market has changed. They must quickly adopt a retention perspective. By focusing attention and events at current customers, their loyalty, longevity, and profitability can be increased.

Aftermarketing Tactics

Aftermarketing is comprised of seven tested tactics to help satisfy and retain customers.

Establishing and Maintaining a Customer Information File

Marketers from the local video store to giants like Kraft General Foods, Pepsico, and R.J. Reynolds are investing millions of dollars in identifying their customers. Their ultimate goals are to avoid the waste and inefficiencies inherent in reaching their customers through the mass media. In some cases, they even consider direct distribution to customers' homes (e.g., KGF's Gevalia coffee and Carnation's Perform pet food).

Blueprinting Customer Contacts

Using a schematic procedure, marketers can identify points of interaction with customers, describing which employees participate in the contact and the nature of the interaction. Such plans can be used to increase satisfaction with these important "moments of truth."

Analyzing Customer Feedback

Read your mail! Customer contacts with a firm should not only be routinely responded to, but also should be treated as a source of important information. This correspondence can be content-analyzed to provide a good report on the nature of customer satisfactions and dissatisfactions. And organizations should respond to compliments as well as complaints.

Conducting Customer Satisfaction Surveys

J.D. Power's various syndicated satisfaction surveys continue to be cited in automobile advertising, but most automakers have sophisticated satisfaction measurement programs of their own in place. For example, it has been reported that Ford Motor Company talks with 2.5 million owners a year to invite reactions to car features and designs.

Formulating and Managing Communication Programs

Outbound communications with customers by a proprietary magazine or newsletter is another way to bond customers to an organization. Over 50 different U.S. marketers in categories as diverse as swimming pool chemicals (Olin Company), overnight courier services (Federal Express), and farm equipment (Deere & Co.) are currently devoting substantial resources to communicating with customers through well-written publications with useful features and only a modicum of sell.

Hosting Special Customer Events or Programs

Customers appreciate events that make them feel special, celebrating their customership with a marketer. For marketers whose products or services offer special cachet, the ability to associate with the marketer might be even more profound. For example, Rolls-Royce hosts owner get-togethers, American Express makes theatrical and other special events available to its Gold Card members, Cellular One holds "tune-up clinics" for cellular telephone subscribers.

Identifying and Reclaiming Lost Customers

Lost customers represent a marketer's mistakes and are often set aside and quickly forgotten. But the reality is that lost customers represent one of the best sources for "new" customers. They know the marketer and the quality of the marketer's products and services and often will return if only invited to do so. MCI has already converted some of its conquest sales offices into win-back and retention centers, where telemarketers' responsibilities include preventing sign-offs and reclaiming lost customers.

Each of these activities can help to increase the likelihood a customer will remain loyal to an organization. And aftermarketing is just as appropriate for the small business as for large multinationals. Anyone who has customers should practice the five A's of aftermarketing:

- **Acquainting** themselves with their customers, getting to know them and their purchasing behavior and needs, identifying high-value customers.

- **Acknowledging** their customers, showing them they are known personally. Also, any communication originated by customers must be acknowledged.

- **Appreciating** their customers and the business they provide. They have numerous other sources and suppliers to chooose from, so it's important to tell them their business is appreciated.

- **Analyzing** the information customers provide in their communications and correspondence. Each contact can provide valuable insights into customers' opinions and feelings.

- **Acting** on what is learned from customers, showing a willingness to listen and a readiness to change operating procedures or products to better satisfy them.

–32–
FREQUENCY MARKETING

Making the Most of Your Customer Base

Richard G. Barlow

Richard G. Barlow is the Founder and President of Frequency Marketing Inc., a marketing agency specializing in the development and implementation of marketing programs aimed at improving customer retention and enhancing share of customer. He is also the publisher of *COLLOQUY*, a quarterly frequency marketing journal produced by Frequency Marketing Inc.

Frequency marketing, also known as loyalty marketing, relationship marketing, and customer marketing, refers to the category of marketing strategies that have as their primary objectives retaining current high-value customers and increasing those customers' purchases over time. The strategies use a variety of value-added offers to attract desirable customers into active, sustainable relationships with the sponsor. Usually characterized by database-driven, systematic, interactive communications between the customer and the sponsor, the strategies typically use direct mail and toll-free telephone access. One commonly accepted working definition of frequency marketing reflects those characteristics:

> To identify, maintain and increase the yield from Best Customers, through long-term, interactive, value-added relationships.[1]

Examples of frequency marketing include a broad variety of marketing programs, ranging from the frequent-flyer and frequent-guest programs that permeate the travel industry to the preferred-customer programs emerging in retailing.

Origins of Frequency Marketing

Although the term *frequency marketing* derives from the frequent-flyer programs beginning in 1981, the origins of this loyalty-focused approach can be found in the trading-stamp programs that flourished most recently in the 1950s and 1960s and in earlier marketing promotions such as the various Ovaltine children's clubs, which used existing media—radio, network television, and direct mail—to establish ongoing relationships with customers. As post–World War II America's economy expanded, however, mass media options proliferated, offering continuously broader reach for advertising. The emerging mass market environment was dominated by a preoccupation with customer acquisition.

When the U.S. economy slowed in the 1970s and 1980s and technological advances in data processing and telecommunications created new opportunities to communicate with customers individually, marketers began to reconsider the potential for building sales through programs aimed at current customers rather

Futurescope

Retaining high-value customers will be increasingly vital in the competitive environment of the 21st century. Marketers now using frequency-marketing programs will need to take advantage of emerging database technologies to continuously adapt to changing customer needs and preferences. New information systems will enable marketers to target individual customer needs with greater sophistication.

than new customers. In certain industries, demand stagnated or declined. At the same time, an intensifying focus on quality produced consumer-perceived brand parity in many categories. As a result, fiercely competitive situations have developed in which customer retention and share of customer have emerged as foremost priorities.

Frequent-Flyer Programs

The launch of the frequent-flyer programs in May 1981 demonstrated these trends in action. American Airlines led the way with its ground-breaking American AAdvantage® program. Deregulation of the airline industry had previously opened up new opportunities for airlines to compete for growth. At the same time, air travel was perceived by the business traveler as a commodity. In the late 1970s, American Airlines and other carriers has already begun to experiment with formalized programs using special recognition and communications to cultivate high-value customers. The AAdvantage program, for example, grew out of an earlier effort, VIT (Very Important Traveler), through which American had identified approximately 250,000 frequent flyers and offered recognition and special treatment.

Tracking individual travel activity was cumbersome, however, until American's computerized SABRE reservations system database provided a simple and accurate way to track mileage (the precise air travel distance flown on American by each enrolled traveler) and limit liability through capacity controls (the number of free "award" seats made available on any given flight). This technological advance permitted the airlines to move from recognition to reward, offering free or discounted air travel and special treatment to its most valuable customers.[2]

Within a week, United Airlines matched American by announcing its own frequent-flyer program, Mileage Plus®, and soon all other U.S. carriers copied the leaders. By 1992, the leading frequent-flyer programs' memberships had grown beyond 15 million travelers each and were continuing to grow by more than 200,000 net new members every month. Top airline marketing executives confirm that, once the initial systems investments were made, frequent-flyer programs became extremely cost-effective, replacing the costly and much less effective mass media approaches to reaching business travelers.

Using actual member travel history, airlines can send customized, personalized marketing messages through the mail announcing new routes, promoting off-season travel, or offering competitive price and bonus frequent-flyer mileage inducements to protect share of customer. By 1983, hotels and car rental companies began to follow the airlines' lead, inviting high-value customers to enroll for special treatment and rewards, based on purchase activity automatically tracked by computerized systems.

Frequency Programs in Other Markets

Other companies, particularly credit card issuers, retailers, and long-distance telephone companies, created customer-retention and share-of-customer strategies based on enhanced special recognition and services for special customers, offering added value through discounts on other companies' products and services. American Express led the way with a variety of innovative services, usually stratified by customer type: Green Card versus Gold Card versus Platinum Card. Extended warranty offers were included for all "cardmembers." Gold Cardmembers got access to special blocks of tickets for plays, concerts, and other events. Platinum Cardmembers got access to events designed for and available only to them.

Retailers like Neiman-Marcus (InCircle® and NM Plus®), Saks Fifth Avenue (Saks First), Sears (Sears Best Customer, Craftsman Club), Kmart (Preferred Reader®, through its specialty chains such as Waldenbooks), and Egghead Software® (CUE) offer preferred customers special discounts, private sales, free services, special financing terms, priority attention, and even free merchandise, based on purchase behavior. Such frequency-marketing programs produce initial sales increases from participating customers in excess of 10 percent and research has shown they account for sustainable incremental sales of approximately that same amount.

What differentiates all frequency programs from offer-driven traditional direct marketing, event-driven sales promotion, and prize-driven continuity schemes is the priority focus on relationship building over the long term. Using rewards, recognition, and special treatment to involve high-value customers in an ongoing dialogue, these programs seek to "turn customers into members,"[3] who then willingly collaborate with the sponsor in the continuing marketing process. With these collaborative relationships[4] established, customers become "insiders," ready and willing to contribute their time, opinions, and discretionary purchase volume in favor of the sponsor.

Basic Elements of Frequency Marketing

Frequency-marketing programs share the following five common elements:

1. A **database** to track purchase activity and maintain other relevant customer information

2. A **format** or structure for establishing and maintaining the relationship with the customer

3. The **benefits** or added value designed to attract the customer into the relationship and maintain his or her commitment

4. The **communications** with the customer, designed to interact with the customer, sending and receiving information

5. The ongoing **analysis** of the program, designed to refine the program in accord with customer preferences

Database

The availability of inexpensive, compact, flexible data-processing equipment and software permits frequency marketers to collect, store, and relate tremendous amounts of information about individual customers. By 1993, most frequency-marketing programs were still using only a minor portion of the broad range of marketing possibilities available through the creative and aggressive application of database technology. Few had gone beyond identifying customers by purchase-volume levels or elementary transactional data such as travel destinations and city pairs in travel marketing and merchandise purchase categories in retailing. The addition of individual demographic, lifestyle, life cycle, and purchase-intention information enhances frequency marketers' ability to individualize their marketing messages and strengthen their relationships with customers.

Format

Every frequency-marketing program requires a format or structure for the relationship between the sponsor and the customer. The most common format is a point structure (frequent flyer, frequent guest), in which customers earn and accumulate a promotional currency (miles, points, etc.), which is redeemable for travel, merchandise, special services, or privileges. Other formats include plateau structures (Neiman-Marcus InCircle), in which purchase-volume levels are designated as goals, the attainment of which triggers rewards or privileges, and simple membership (Preferred Reader, Sears Best Customer), in which every member receives a list of benefits as part of his or her membership.

Benefits

Benefits represent the added value used to involve customers in the special relationships marketers seek to establish through frequency-marketing programs. They are not always intrinsic to the sponsor's product or service and can be classified as either "soft benefits" or "hard benefits." Soft benefits include special recognition and treatment, such as frequent-flyer upgrades, special check-in lines, special discounts, private sales, and free services. Hard benefits include free trips, free merchandise, or free entertainment events that the sponsor purchases or for which the customer would otherwise have to pay personally. Most research shows that soft benefits are more effective in sustaining loyalty over time, although hard benefits are necessary to attract customers initially.

Communications

The most effective frequency-marketing programs maintain regular, frequent communications with customers, usually through a periodic newsletter or bulletin, through toll-free telephone access, and through special surveys, events, and face-to-face contact. In general, the customer's sense of commitment and involvement in the program varies in direct relation to the amount and relevance of the communication he or she exchanges with the sponsor. Personalized, customized newsletters and mailers are well-received and well-read. Surveys elicit high response rates. Toll-free phone calls are packed with usable marketing information volunteered by collaborative customers.

Analysis

Frequency-marketing programs are highly measurable in their impact, precise and accurate down to the individual customer level, and they provide a real-time customer research mechanism capable of directing virtually every aspect of product and marketing strategy. The most successful programs involve a systematic approach to ongoing analysis of results and customer feedback.

Notes

1. Trademark, Frequency Marketing, Inc., Cincinnati, Ohio, 1993.

2. "A Candid Conversation with Frequent-Flyer Pioneer Mike Gunn of American Airlines," *COLLOQUY,* 3, no. 2 (Frequency Marketing, Inc., 1992).

3. Rosabeth Moss Kanter, "From the Editor," *Harvard Business Review* (January-February 1991).

4. Don Peppers and Martha Rogers, Ph.D., *The One to One Future* (New York: Currency Doubleday, 1993), pp. 51–94.

–33–
MARKETING TRAINING BEYOND 2000

Richard J. Chvala

Richard J. Chvala serves as an adjunct professor at the University of Richmond School of Business Management. He is Senior Consultant, Sales and Marketing Training, for Ethyl Corporation, a *Fortune* 500 company based in Richmond, Virginia. Chvala also serves on the national board of the American Marketing Association, and was the keynote speaker at the AMA's First International Congress on Customer Satisfaction. Rich has more than 15 years of experience as a national sales manager and marketing executive for both capital goods and service companies. Chvala's training specialties include strategic selling, customer communications, and creating value for the customer. He is the co-author of *Total Quality and Marketing*. Chvala received his undergraduate degree in biochemistry from Michigan Technological University and his M.B.A. from Michigan.

Stu Leonard, the now-famous Connecticut grocer idolized by Tom Peters, states that he "simply hires nice people" to assure customer satisfaction for his shoppers. Unfortunately, all life's tasks are not as simple as checking out groceries; nor can you expect people to remain "nice" long after they are employed. So what can a company do to remain competitive in these fast-paced, turbulent times?

Many companies—over 37 percent of the *Fortune* 500, according to a 1992 American Society of Training and Development (ASTD) study—have invested in marketing training to keep their personnel motivated and skilled to succeed in the eyes of the customer. More than $240 million was spent on marketing training for U.S. companies in 1992. What did this among of money provide in terms of skills development, and where is marketing training headed into the next century?

Most marketing training conducted today falls under three guidelines:

• Employee orientation to the markets served

• Skills training for sales, marketing, and customer-service personnel

• Training to promote a cultural change toward improved market orientation

The ASTD conducts benchmark studies of a company's training program to determine what impact it has on the bottom line. Training programs are evaluated to determine the level of value that training has on the culture and profitability of a company.

Good training programs must provide the participant with a level of understanding that can be put to use to make a difference in his or her position. Most companies today use customer satisfaction surveys to determine whether a training program has had a positive impact. Accountability in marketing training can also be measured by studying trends in margin or market share.

Fundamentally, what marketing training does today is to provide companies with a fast-paced, mini-M.B.A. that is relevant to the immediate and future skills

Futurescope

Future marketing training will involve customers and suppliers along with a company's employees as they study market trends and establish processes that better serve those markets. Partnerships will involve suppliers on through to end-users, as well as regulatory agencies, to combat the competitive pacts that are evolving in many global regions. The 21st century will be a faster-paced, more competitive world, with a greater need for reliable information and, most importantly, employees who can react successfully in implementing a successful strategy to satisfy customers. That reason alone is why marketing training will be all the more necessary after the year 2000.

needed by their employees. Look to these areas of marketing training to be the fads in global companies at the turn of the century.

- Establishing relationships with suppliers and governments
- Joint marketing strategies with customers
- Immediate market research through "telesurveys"
- Competitive analysis systems for all employees
- Supplier-customer generated pricing strategies
- Selling to supply chain–managed customers
- Negotiating 20-year supply contracts the "win-win" way
- Team marketing—internal customer service
- Employees as distributor channels

Gaining the Edge with Marketing Training

Training in marketing runs the gamut from simple communication techniques and understanding different personalities, all the way to sophisticated marketing research equations such as multivariate beta coefficients in multiple regressions. Obviously, one needs to evaluate what level of marketing training would best benefit the population being trained.

John Akers, the IBM chairman who stepped down in 1993 during IBM's doldrums, stated that a primary reason for IBM's market share loss was not IBM's lack of product diversity, but rather "our lack of focusing on the customer and training our people in the care and handling of customers."

A benchmark study by ASTD concluded that 37 percent of *Fortune* 500 companies spent nearly $240 million in 1992 conducting marketing training for their personnel and distributors. What is this great endeavor, marketing training, and will it benefit you and your company in today's fast-paced, competitive environment?

Can marketing training really make a difference in a large corporation? In 1987, a large customer of Richmond-based Ethyl Corporation (*Fortune* 200, $3.0 billion in chemical and pharmaceutical sales) called the company "slow and arrogant in its treatment of customers." In 1991, that same customer awarded Ethyl its "Supplier of the Decade" award. Here's how Ethyl used marketing training to change its culture.

Ethyl's training program used a process that satisfies the needs of both the organization and the individual. Given today's competitive market environment and often competitive internal environment, this is no small feat. This process can help your company to determine what marketing training is valuable and to establish a system of training modules that support your company's goals.

Steps to Reaching Your Company's Vision Through Marketing Training

The CEO Must Take an Active Role and Champion the Efforts

In 1988, several marketing managers, representing most of Ethyl's operating divisions, met to discuss how to change the company's culture to be more market-oriented. This group requested the CEO of Ethyl, Bruce C. Gottwald, to assist them in reaching the goal of creating a stronger customer focus throughout the corporation. He agreed that the cultural shift was needed and volunteered to lend his prestige and energy to the effort.

Appoint a Team or Committee of Cross-Functional Personnel to Identify and Act on Necessary Changes

During that session in 1988, a steering group was formed that became known as the Ethyl Marketing Forum. This group was made up of marketing, sales, manufacturing, R&D, logistics, and administrative personnel representing Ethyl's chemicals, plastics, pharmaceutical, and insurance divisions. This team became the steering force for the cultural change effort.

Perform a Benchmark, Image, or Customer-Satisfaction Survey or Market Review

Over the course of that year, Marketing Forum members conducted several appraisals, both internally and externally, of Ethyl's status as a market-oriented company. Customers, vendors, competitors, and Ethyl employees were asked to evaluate Ethyl on a number of parameters, detailing both the effectiveness of our marketing and customer satisfaction with our products and services.

Insist That the Team Listen to Outsiders

It is difficult for chemical engineers and Ph.D. chemists to value the input of nontechnical people. However, in our evaluation process, we listened to other chemical companies, as well as leading spokespersons on several subjects relative to improving our market focus. Predispositions and biases were subordinated whenever possible.

Identify the Changes Required

The Marketing Forum developed a laundry list of needed improvements, ranging from the telephone systems used at division headquarters sites and substantial changes in the organizational structure, all the way to adjustments in the corporate portfolio of businesses. This list, known as the Marketing Forum Priority Areas, included data systems (laptops) for field sales personnel, establishing a market research group, greater emphasis on strategic planning, a new integrated planning process, and refocusing the Chemicals group to serve existing and new markets with higher levels of service.

Set Up a Timetable

Change does not pace itself, and a sense of urgency sometimes creates the necessary environment for change. Ethyl Corporation has a long history of financial success, so the company was not looking at change to reverse a downward trend, but possibly even more important, to maintain positive growth through the turbulent 1990s. The Marketing Forum established an aggressive agenda designed to train all employees in multiple facets of market awareness and to conduct marketing skills training for over 450 salaried personnel.

Assemble a Training Calendar to Implement the Improvement of Skills

The corporate training organization enlisted several training and consultant groups to design and deliver a 14-course curriculum of sales, marketing, and customer-service workshops over a period of four years. After the initial training period of 3–4 years, many of these programs are now offered to new employees or serve to maintain the skills levels of experienced personnel. A number of Ethyl's customers request that these courses be offered to their employees as well, making the marketing training program a significant added value to customers.

Communicate Each Step of the Path to All Employees

Scheduled communication of our progress toward an improved market focus was delivered via executive speeches, company newsletter, computer mail messages, and a quarterly, company-wide video program. This communication effort kept the process at the forefront of people's priorities and made the transition easier.

Use a Non-Political, Diplomatic Facilitator to Keep the Effort Focused

A task as ambitious as changing a corporation's culture is not a part-time occupation. Also, some top-level executives might have seen this movement as a challenge to their power base. Therefore, it is best to assign someone who can accomplish large-scale tasks without a built-in power base. This person serves best by not personally seeking rewards within the organization (i.e., promotions, transfers, etc.).

Employ Outsiders
(Recognized Consultants, Esteemed Professors, Etc.)
When the Going Gets Tough

Ethyl engaged notable proponents to seek a following on several key issues: Michael Porter on the value of good competitive analysis, Philip Kotler on marketing planning, professors of the Fuqua School, Duke University, for an executive marketing program, and EMME Associates for sales skills training. Outsiders can shed a different, perhaps more objective light on situations that might be viewed from only one angle by internal personnel.

Reward Those Who Change

Most people are willing to change and to improve on and expand their abilities when they discover that without change, they might be left at the back of the pack. Of the 18 individuals who made up the initial Marketing Forum, 16 were promoted into director, general manager, or vice president positions within the company.

Identify, Lower, or Remove Barriers
That Slow the Process

Authority levels, cross-functional communications, non-sales customer contact, and a telemarketing function are examples of areas that endured substantial change in Ethyl's quest for an improved market orientation.

Don't Tell Your Customers That Change
Has Occurred Until the Change Is Debugged
and Effective Throughout the Company

Nothing can slow the process more than to have a customer telling you that "nothing has happened" or "I don't see what you are saying." Customers as well as employees will interpret firsthand the changes that your company has undergone far better than reading about it in an advertisement.

Be Proud of Your Success

If you improve substantially, throw a party and reward all participants and contributors, customers and employees alike.

—34—
ETHICS BUILDS TRUST IN MARKETING RELATIONSHIPS

O. C. Ferrell

O. C. Ferrell is Interim Dean and Distinguished Professor of Marketing and Business Ethics in the Fogelman College of Business and Economics at The University of Memphis. Dr. Ferrell was chairman of the American Marketing Association Ethics Committee that developed the current AMA Code of Ethics. He has published articles on marketing ethics in the *Journal of Marketing, Journal of Marketing Research, Journal of Business Research, Journal of Macromarketing, Journal of the Academy of Marketing Science, Journal of Advertising, Human Relations, Journal of Business Ethics,* as well as others. He has co-authored ten textbooks including a leading basic marketing text, *Marketing: Concepts and Strategies,* Ninth Edition, and *Business Ethics: Ethical Decision Making and Cases,* Second Edition, and a tradebook, *In Pursuit of Ethics.*

Ethics is a key concern in daily customer and employee relationships. Ethical marketing decisions foster trust, which holds buyer-seller relationships together. Ethical transgressions destroy trust and make continuing business difficult, if not impossible. A recent Roper Organization poll found that 38 percent of adults up to the age of 30 say that corruption and deceit are necessary for getting ahead. Therefore, companies must create an ethical climate and be vigilant in protecting their interests from individuals who are anxious to take advantage.

Companies should take an ethical position and establish marketing policies on ethics. Often employees don't have enough experience in business to know the right decision when confronted with an ethics-related dilemma. Employees are most likely to look at managers and co-workers for signals on how to behave when confronted with the opportunity to take advantage of a situation or to determine what is right or wrong.

Having good personal ethics is necessary but insufficient to make the right decisions at work. Marketers who come to work well-equipped with personal ethics might not know how to apply their beliefs to complex marketing issues. Surveys show that the majority of people will follow the directions they are given and will make unethical decisions if management policy makes such actions appear necessary. Sears' Chairman, Ed Brennan, took responsibility for employees' overcharging auto repair customers. He eliminated incentive compensation and goal-setting systems for Sears' automotive service advisers who tried to meet sales quotas on products like shock absorbers. Too often, employees will do what it takes to meet sales quotas or goals set by management.

No one has yet discovered a universally accepted approach to marketing ethics, but failure to address ethics and develop policies and guidelines to resolve issues compounds the problem. A Dallas-based retailer with 75 stores lost millions of dollars in settling a lawsuit because there were no store policies on selling dangerous products to children. One child is permanently incapacitated both mentally and physically from inhaling a pressurized substance from a can purchased at the store.

Futurescope

Ethics will remain a key aspect of marketing in the 21st century, as collaborative relationships based on trust form the central type of marketing partnerships. Moreover, litigation will sustain its current rate of increase, meaning that profound financial consequences will stem from unethical conduct. The internationalization of business will further complicate ethical matters as executives from various cultural backgrounds strive to harmonize their viewpoints of acceptable marketing practices.

Figure 1 American Marketing Association Code of Ethics

Members of the American Marketing Association (AMA) are committed to ethical professional conduct. They have joined together in subscribing to this Code of Ethics embracing the following topics.

Responsibilities of the Marketer

Marketers must accept responsibility for the consequences of their activities and make every effort to ensure that their decisions, recommendations, and actions function to identify, serve, and satisfy all relevant publics: consumers, organizations and society. Marketers' professional conduct must be guided by:

1. The basic rule of professional ethics: not knowingly to do harm;

2. The adherence to all applicable laws and regulations;

3. The accurate representation of their education, training and experience; and

4. The active support, practice and promotion of this Code of Ethics.

Honesty and Fairness

Marketers shall uphold and advance the integrity, honor, and dignity of the marketing profession by:

1. Being honest in serving consumers, clients, employees, suppliers, distributors and the public;

2. Not knowingly participating in conflict of interest without prior notice to all parties involved; and

3. Establishing equitable fee schedules including the payment or receipt of usual, customary and/or legal compensation for marketing exchanges.

Rights and Duties of Parties

Participants in the marketing exchange process should be able to expect that:

1. Products and services offered are safe and fit for their intended uses;

2. Communications about offered products and services are not deceptive;

3. All parties intend to discharge their obligations, financial and otherwise, in good faith; and

4. Appropriate internal methods exist for equitable adjustment and/or redress of grievances concerning purchases.

It is understood that the above would include, *but is not limited to,* the following responsibilities of the marketer:

In the area of product development management:

Disclosure of all substantial risks associated with product or service usage

Identification of any product component substitution that might materially change the product or impact on the buyer's purchase decision

Identification of extra-cost added features

In the area of promotions:

Avoidance of false and misleading advertising

Rejection of high pressure manipulations, or misleading sales tactics

Avoidance of sales promotions that use deception or manipulation

In the area of distribution:

Not manipulating the availability of a product for purpose of exploitation

Not using coercion in the marketing channel

Not exerting undue influence over the resellers' choice to handle a product

In the area of pricing:

Not engaging in price fixing

Not practicing predatory pricing

Disclosing the full price associated with any purchase

In the area of marketing research:

Prohibiting selling or fund raising under the guise of conducting research

Maintaining research integrity by avoiding misrepresentation and omission of pertinent research data

Treating outside clients and suppliers fairly

Organizational Relationships

Marketers should be aware of how their behavior may influence or impact on the behavior of others in organizational relationships. They should not encourage or apply coercion to obtain unethical behavior in their relationships with others, such as employees, suppliers or customers.

1. Apply confidentiality and anonymity in professional relationships with regard to privileged information.

2. Meet their obligations and responsibilities in contracts and mutual agreements in a timely manner.

3. Avoid taking the work of others, in whole, or in part, and represent this work as their own or directly benefit from it without compensation or consent of the originator or owner.

4. Avoid manipulation to take advantage of situations to maximize personal welfare in a way that unfairly deprives or damages the organization or others.

Any AMA members found to be in violation of any provision of this Code of Ethics may have his or her Association membership suspended or revoked.

Source: Reprinted by permission of the American Marketing Association.

The store ignored the drug abuse concerns of the local community and sold the product to the child.

Not only do large corporations have to deal with ethical issues, but even the smallest family business needs coherent policies for marketing ethics. A small business can be lulled into thinking ethics is something learned at home; they don't want to appear to preach. Leadership is needed because there will be differences of opinion on what to do. Letting each employee establish ethical policy for the company is asking for trouble. Michael Milken established his own brand of ethics and today, his former employer, Drexel, Burnham, Lambert, is out of business.

Top management cannot always tell employees exactly what to do, but top management can provide general guidelines and direction to eliminate major ethical mistakes. For example, managers can provide directives to subordinates to disclose risks associated with products or information regarding the function, value, or use of the product. Additional efforts can be made to control bribes, deceptive sales techniques, price fixing, and sexual harassment and discrimination.

Unless a company develops and enforces some standards or policies to ensure proper ethical behavior, the marketers are always taking a risk that a few individuals will make an unethical decision and cause serious problems for the company. Employees need to be free to come forward when they believe they are being asked to do something unethical. Marketing managers have to develop an ethically correct organizational climate where employees feel free to talk. If you destroy openness, you destroy the ability to be an ethically responsible company.

Almost everyone who works is faced with tough ethical choices daily. Many companies, such as Citicorp, Hershey Foods, and Ford Motor Co., are conducting ethics training programs and developing policies to improve their ethics. If a company has not addressed ethical concerns, it is in danger of losing the trust of both its employees and customers. It is impossible to remain competitive when trust is broken.

Codes of ethics are formalized rules and standards that describe what marketers should expect of each other. Codes of ethics encourage ethical behavior by eliminating opportunities for unethical behavior, because expectations and punishment for violating rules are clearly defined. Codes of ethics are not so detailed that they take into account every situation, but they should provide general guidelines for achieving organizational goals and objectives in an ethically acceptable manner. The American Marketing Association Code of Ethics appears in Figure 1. This code does not cover every ethical issue related to marketing, but it is a useful overview of what marketers believe are sound moral principles for guiding marketing activities. The code could be used to help structure a marketing organization's code of ethics.

—35—
IMPROVING MARKETING PRODUCTIVITY

Jagdish N. Sheth and Rajendra S. Sisodia

Dr. Jagdish N. Sheth is the Charles Kellstadt Professor of Marketing at Emory University. Formerly, he ws the Robert Brooker Professor of Marketing at the University of Southern California and the Walter Stellner Distinguished Professor of Marketing at the University of Illinois. Dr. Sheth has published numerous books and articles in marketing and other business disciplines and has received numerous awards for his work, including the P.D. Converse Award from the American Marketing Association.

Dr. Rajendra S. Sisodia is Associate Professor of Business at George Mason University in Fairfax, Virginia. Before joining GMU, he was Assistant Professor of Marketing at Boston University. Dr. Sisodia has an M. Phil. and a Ph.D. in Marketing and Business Policy from Columbia University. His research, teaching and consulting expertise spans the areas of marketing strategy and business impacts of information technology. Dr. Sisodia has published over forty articles in conference proceedings and journals such as *Harvard Business Review* and *Journal of Business Strategy.*

It is generally acknowledged, even among those inclined to extol the virtues of the "good old days," that businesses today deliver greater value to the typical customer than they did in the past. A greater variety of higher quality products and services is now more conveniently available at reasonable prices to almost every customer. Much of the credit for this happier state is certainly attributable to the ascendancy of the marketing function in the modern corporation. After all, it was the "marketing concept" that first articulated a vision of the customer as the defining purpose of business and the determinant of corporate success. However, the marketing function in many companies has come to consume a disproportionately high share of corporate resources, inviting intense scrutiny from corporate cost-cutters. Further, there appears, at macro level, to be a low correlation between the level of spending on marketing and measures of overall financial performance and competitive position. Many firms are getting a low to negative return on incremental marketing spending. These factors have focused renewed attention on the critical issue of marketing productivity.

The Productivity Crisis in Marketing

In the quest for greater efficiency, other functional areas within business have undergone fundamental, frequently wrenching, change:

- Manufacturing has become substantially more efficient (through automation, just-in-time techniques, product redesign for assembly and manufacture, flexible manufacturing systems, and so on) and more quality-focused. As a rough estimate, manufacturing now accounts for about 30 percent of total corporate costs, down from approximately 50 percent after World War II.

- Management (defined here to include finance, accounting, human resources, and support functions such as legal departments, as well as R&D) has raised its efficiency through "downsizing," "rightsizing," outsourcing, and business

---

Futurescope

The quest for greater productivity has finally reached marketing departments. While some marketers, using old "tried and true" approaches, are facing a crisis, innovative practitioners are meeting the challenge. With a more comprehensive approach to productivity—effective efficiency—marketers using better measurement techniques, more sensible strategies, and more effective systems of monitoring and evaluating productivity will win the day.

process reengineering. The share of corporate costs attributable to management have fallen from 30 percent to 20 percent.

• That leaves about 50 percent for marketing (up from 20 percent), including the cost of selling, distribution, advertising, sales promotion, customer service, etc.

Marketing's importance—along with the size of its budgets—has increased as companies have faced higher levels of competition in increasingly global markets. Its exalted status as the generator of corporate revenues, profitability, and visibility has tended to shield it from the deep cuts other departments have endured in the past decade. Indeed, though marketing is the biggest *discretionary* spending area in most companies, it is also the area to which many companies wish they could devote even more resources. This situation, we strongly believe, will not persist. In fact, there are clear signs already that CEOs are demanding a higher level of accountability from marketing than ever before.

The Changes, the Responses, and the New "Rules"

Marketing efficiency was relatively high when the consumer market was homogeneous and mass media were dominant. Many basic needs had not yet been met, and the intensity of competition (certainly from global competitors) was much lower. All of these conditions are now the exception rather than the rule.

Marketing's response to the tremendously heightened competitive intensity of the past few decades was twofold. The first was to increase expenditures on virtually every aspect of marketing, from greater and more frequent discounting to more pervasive advertising to intensified selling efforts. The second was to proliferate greater variety in products, in prices, in distribution channels, and so on. Each of these actions, while perhaps justifiable in isolation and for short-run considerations, contributed to making the marketing function increasingly unwieldy and expensive.

CEOs are now subjecting the marketing function to an unprecedented level of critical scrutiny. There is an increasingly widespread belief that all these marketing dollars are being poorly used, sometimes even to the detriment of the business they are supporting. For example, Fred Webster of Dartmouth interviewed the CEOS of 30 major corporations to determine their views of the marketing function.[1] Two of the four key areas of concern were the diminishing productivity of marketing expenditures and a poor understanding of the financial implications of marketing actions. A third concern—a lack of innovation and entrepreneurial thinking—also relates to marketing's failure to address the productivity issue in new ways.

. . . the major issue is one of marketing productivity. Marketing needs a better method of making cost/benefit analysis on marketing expenditures— to make good, intelligent choices on how to get the most out of our marketing dollars, including marketing support, not just research on new products, media, et cetera . . . the concern is that while costs are rising, marketing is not finding new ways to improve marketing efficiency.[2]

While the comments from CEOs and consulting firms are quite broad, we can provide some particulars:

- Many companies today practice "Just-in-Time" manufacturing but "Just-in-Case" marketing. By this we mean that companies are failing to adequately leverage their efficient demand-driven production systems by coupling them with similar marketing systems. They continue to practice forecast-driven marketing. The data on this are clear: between 1982 and 1993, manufacturers reduced their inventory levels dramatically, from 2.0 times monthly sales to around 1.4 times monthly sales currently. By contract, retail and wholesale inventories have actually risen in the same time period.[3]

- Packaged goods manufacturers spent $6.1 billion on over 300 billion coupons in 1993. Of these, only 1.8 percent were redeemed, and of those, 80 percent were redeemed by shoppers who would have bought the brand anyway.[4] Of the other 20 percent, many are redeemed by shoppers who are pure deal seekers and are unlikely to ever purchase the brand without a large incentive.

- Likewise, it has been estimated that excessive trade promotions add about $20 billion a year to the grocery bills of U.S. consumers. Much of this is due to the practice of "forward buying." As a result, it takes an average of 84 days for a product to get from the manufacturer to the consumer.

These few examples illustrate the kinds of productivity problems that characterize marketing today. Before we can address these problems, we believe it is important to adopt a broader view of marketing productivity.

An Expanded Concept of Marketing Productivity: Effective Efficiency

The marketing function traditionally was viewed as inherently inefficient, given its domain and the nature of its objectives and tools. A long-standing belief also has been that it is difficult, indeed almost impossible, to accurately measure marketing efficiency and productivity. For example, in 1948, Nil Houston of the Harvard Business School wrote in his dissertation, ". . . a quantitative assessment of the efficiency of marketing cannot be made."[5]

The early emphasis in trying to improve marketing efficiency, predominantly to attempt to minimize marketing costs, was driven by the recognized difficulty of adequately measuring the output of marketing. It was also due to an implicit belief that marketing did not create value in any tangible sense and hence was an activity on which the minimum necessary amount of resources should be expended. In his seminal dissertation on the subject, Robert Buzzel vigorously challenged this belief, and today we have ample evidence that judiciously expended marketing resources can be tremendously productive.[6] For example, the return on a dollar of advertising for AT&T's early "Reach out and touch someone" campaign (when it still had a dominant market share in the long distance telecommunications market) was estimated to be over four dollars! John Little's advocacy in the late 1970s of "response reporting" was mainly in this spirit; by determining the elasticity of sales and profits to various marketing stimuli, marketing resources could be expended in a highly productive manner.

As Buzzell pointed out, marketing does not produce anything; it performs functions *around* goods and services. This makes marketing productivity very difficult to measure. Further, many functions performed by marketing may over time become sufficiently routine that they become absorbed into other functional areas. For example, many food products used to be sold in bulk to retailers, who would then sell to customers in smaller packages. When manufacturers began shipping their products in multiple sizes, a marketing function became a manufacturing function. Over time, this type of shift can cause marketing productivity to appear to be diminishing. However, most such manufacturing changes are initiated by marketing, and this "problem" will become even more acute as more companies adopt "mass customization" approaches to manufacturing, with many of marketing's value-added activities being performed by manufacturing.

The Need for Better Measurement

Notwithstanding these challenges, we believe there is so much to be gained from improvements in marketing productivity that even imperfect measurements can be of great value. To a degree, we subscribe to the assertion "You cannot improve what you cannot measure." Specifically, we believe that we must measure the right things; otherwise, our attempts at improvement will, by definition, be misdirected.

Traditionally, productivity has been measured in terms of the *quantity* of output for a given amount of input. However, such measures are unsatisfactory, in that they fail to adjust for changes in the desirability of the output. In an often-cited example, the output of a steel mill is measured in "tons of steel," disregarding the fact that the quality and value-added of such steel may increase substantially over time.

This problem is especially acute for marketing measurements, since marketing deals with so many intangibles. To address it, we suggest that marketing productivity be defined to mean the amount of *desirable* output per unit of input. In other words, output should be measured in terms of quality as well as quantity.

The productivity of a salesperson thus is more than the number of sales calls made or even the number of transactions that result. It also includes the effectiveness of those sales calls (e.g., their long-run impact on the relationship with those customers), the profitability of the resulting transactions, and the impact of today's business mix on the future. Likewise, a productive advertisement could be defined as one that maximizes the quality-adjusted amount of exposure for a given budget.

The desired output of marketing can be stated in simple terms as follows: acquiring and retaining customers profitably. It follows then that a good measure of marketing productivity must include the economics of customer acquisition as well as those of customer retention. We operationalize this as follows:

- For customer acquisition, we propose a measure of the revenues due to marketing actions from new customers, divided by the costs of those actions, adjusted by a Customer Satisfaction Index (CSI). This formulation reflects our belief that new customers must be acquired based on the creation of highly satisfying exchanges, rather than the use of "hard selling" and deceptive advertising. Customers are too often acquired by overpromising and then

Figure 1   Marketing Efficiency and Effectiveness

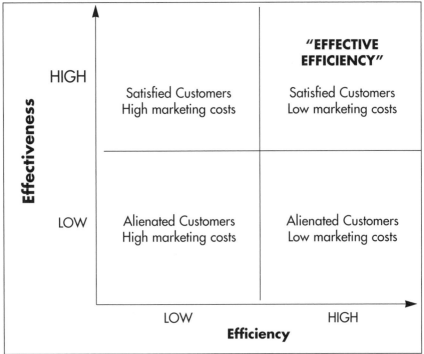

underdelivering on their heightened expectations, which usually leads to customer dissatisfaction. Customer satisfaction measurements are now becoming quite commonplace in many industries. For example, J. D. Power & Associates measures customer satisfaction in the automobile and personal computer industries.

- For customer retention, we adjust the measure of revenues/costs for existing customers by what we term a Customer Loyalty Index (CLI) because customer retention in the long run requires more than the maintenance of high customer satisfaction. Even ostensibly satisfied customers can be induced to switch to a rival offering unless they have been strongly bonded to a firm's offering. The CLI is closely related to the problem of customer "churn" (customers frequently switching between providers based on inducements), which is a significant problem in a number of industries today.

In the broader sense described above, marketing productivity as we define it includes both the dimensions of efficiency (doing things right) as well as effectiveness (doing the right things), as depicted in Figure 1. Ideally, the marketing function should generate satisfied customers at low cost. Too often, however, companies either create satisfied customers at unacceptably high cost or alienate customers (as well as employees) in their search for marketing efficiencies. In far too many cases, the marketing function accomplishes neither.

Marketing needs to pursue the ideal of *effective efficiency* in all of its programs and processes. This ideal guides our identification of the ways in which marketing productivity may be improved.

How Marketing Productivity Can Be Improved

Some part of marketing's productivity problem is simply due to poor marketing. In other words, companies too often fail to apply marketing concepts in a balanced manner. Too many companies, for example, emphasize capturing market share over developing strategies to grow the market—a crucial distinction that leads to misapplied marketing dollars and heavy competitive retaliation. Likewise, many companies demonstrate a poor understanding of how the elements of the marketing mix interrelate and deploy excessive resources on some aspects to the detriment of others. Often, for example, companies fail to see that the "weak link" in their marketing mix may be inadequate market coverage. Consequently, they may squander excessive resources on advertising or on lowering the price.

Beyond correcting such fundamental marketing mistakes, marketing productivity can be improved in a number of other ways. We have identified several approaches, each of which is briefly described below.

Figure 2   Approaches to Improving Marketing Productivity

Better Marketing Accounting

- *Activity-Based Costing:* Understand where resources are being spent, where customer value is being created, and where money is being made or lost.

Greater Use of Collaborative Strategies

- *Partnering:* Treat your suppliers and customers as partners in lowering system-wide costs and adding value.
- *Relationship Marketing:* Be selective about customers, and take a long-term, win-win perspective.
- *Marketing Alliances:* Share resources and opportunities with other companies serving the same customers.

Better Domain Definition

- *Make vs. Buy: Insourcing vs. Outsourcing:* Focus on your marketing core competencies and let outside experts handle the rest.
- *Getting Customers To Do More Work:* Lower costs and increase customer satisfaction by adding customers to the value chain.

Unbundling and Rebundling Services

- Uncover the hiddent costs of free service, and create new revenue sources.

Rationalizing the Marketing Mix

- *Umbrella Branding:* Increase return on branding by developing brand names with broad applicability to multiple products and markets.

- *Rationalizing and Recycling Advertising:* Remove conflicts of interest in agency compensation methods, unbundle advertising creation and placement, and understand advertising life cycles
- *Reducing Product Proliferation:* Variety does not always equate to value; reduce customer confusion and marketing costs by matching product lines with distinct market segments.

Use of Information Technology

- *Data-Based Marketing:* Target marketing efforts more precisely, but ensure that you are creating additional value for the customer and are acutely sensitive to privacy concerns.
- *Front-line Information Systems:* Deploy information tools where they have the greatest impact on customer service and satisfaction: at the front line.
- *Marketing and the Global Information Highway:* Prepare now for a radically different, more integrated mode of marketing in the future, predicated on "total customer convenience."

Better Monitoring and Control

- *Adjusting Compensation of Marketing Personnel:* Compensation drivers must be linked to the need for effective efficiency in all marketing activities.
- *Continuous Assessment of Marketing Practices:* Beware of creeping marketing incrementalism; take a periodic "zero-based" view of marketing practices.

Better Marketing Accounting

As Philip Kotler points out, companies such as General Foods, DuPont, and Johnson & Johnson have established a "marketing controller" position to help improve marketing efficiency.[7] However, this practice is still limited to a few companies and focuses heavily on efficiency of expenditures and profitability. It does not capture the effectiveness dimension. We believe that marketing needs to work with the accounting function to develop a comprehensive marketing accounting discipline.

Developments in this field are occurring rapidly, from the concept of "Economic Value Added" (linking corporate spending to shareholder value creation) to more recent attempts at measuring intellectual capital.[8] These efforts grapple with the measurement of the largely intangible elements that comprise much of the assets and added value of many of today's businesses. While it is beyond the scope of this article to describe these efforts in detail, it is evident that they represent potentially very valuable tools for measuring (and thus improving) marketing productivity.

One accounting tool that is clearly of great importance for marketing is activity-based costing.

Activity-Based Costing (ABC)

According to Robert Kaplan, one of the pioneers in the ABC field:

Failure to (completely) understand cost drivers leads to SKU proliferation; pricing divorced from actual operating costs; poor understanding of product, brand and customer profitability; ineffective vendor relationships; and hidden costs from inefficient processes.[9]

The fundamental question posed through the use of ABC is: "Would the customer pay for this activity if they knew you were doing it?" For many marketing activities, the answer is "No."

Traditional accounting methods allocate overhead as a percentage of direct labor. ABC is based on some fairly simple principles. The first is that since most business activities support the production and delivery of goods and services, they should be regarded as direct product costs. ABC thus abandons the traditional accounting practice of treating large blocks of corporate and overhead expenditures as "fixed costs" allocated evenly across all products. Rather, it defines a much wider section of corporate activities and costs as "variable," allocating them as directly as possible to specific goods and services.

The use of ABC is clearly essential to any attempts to measure marketing productivity. In the grocery business, the use of Direct Product Profitability (DPP) has led to substantial improvements in overall productivity. We suggest that marketing productivity be measured at the account level in a similar way, using a combination of activity-based and account-based costing for marketing activities. Account-based costing would enable companies to eliminate unintended (i.e., hidden) cross-subsidies between accounts which often invite "cream-skimming" competitors to take away highly profitable customers.

The use of ABC in marketing raises efficiency through possible reduction in, as well as more balanced application of, marketing resources.

Greater Use of Collaborative Strategies

A number of collaborative marketing approaches are of particular value in improving marketing productivity. The three that we highlight here are partnering, relationship marketing, and marketing alliances. Each of the three allows for greater resource efficiency, as well as improving customer satisfaction.

Partnering

Dramatic gains in distribution and marketing efficiencies can be achieved when buyers and sellers agree to work together. Such "partnering" between members of a value chain, such as retailers and manufacturers, represents a major departure from their traditionally antagonistic relationship. Both are part of a single process—distributing products to customers—which technology can greatly streamline and simplify.[10] For example, Black & Decker describes its new distribution philosophy as "Sell one, ship one, build one." Inventory is pulled through the system rather than pushed down. Much lower average levels of inventory are coupled with higher levels of product availability for customers.

Partnering enables its practitioners to gain the advantages of vertical integration without the attendant drawbacks. This is sometimes referred to as "virtual integration." Partnering had its roots in the "Quick Response" movement in the apparel industry; in the grocery business, it is known as "Efficient Consumer Response." A report done by Kurt Salmon Associates for the Food Marketing Institute found that ECR has the potential to achieve a 41 percent reduction in inventory and save $30 billion a year in the grocery industry alone.[11] The ECR system is based on timely, accurate, and paperless information flow between suppliers, distributors, retail stores, and consumer households. Its objective is to provide a "smooth, continual product flow matched to consumption." It focuses on the efficiency of the total supply system, rather than on the efficiency of any of its components.

Central to such partnering arrangements are the enabling technologies of bar-coded product identification and electronic data interchange (EDI), along with the reengineering of business processes within and across firms in the value chain. These systems improve efficiencies and customer service primarily by replacing physical assets with information. They reduce the retailer's inventory while providing a supply of merchandise that is closely coordinated with the actual buying patterns of consumers. These systems also allow retailers to make purchase commitments closer to the time of sale. Resources that were earlier tied up in inventory can be deployed elsewhere: to increased advertising, to add new product lines, or to improve the bottom line. The result is a win-win-win outcome. Consumers consistently find the merchandise they want in stock (often at lower prices); suppliers increase sales, lower costs, and cement ties with retailers; and retailers gain increased sales and inventory turns and more satisfied customers.

Retailers such as Wal-Mart, JC Penney, and Dillard's and manufacturers such as VF Corp., Levi Strauss, and Procter & Gamble who have all adopted QR have achieved significant gains in market share and profitability. Further, all of these companies have more satisfied customers as well, since customers are better able to obtain desired merchandise at reasonable prices,

Relationship Marketing

Related to partnering but one step short of it is relationship marketing. Firms are increasingly adopting a relationship marketing mindset in dealing with their customers. By this is meant a long-term, mutually beneficial arrangement in which both the buyer and seller focus on value enhancement through the creation of more satisfying exchanges. At the same time, both buyers and sellers are able to reduce their costs. Buyers do it through reducing their search and transaction costs, while sellers are able to reduce advertising and selling expenses.

Maintaining strong relationships with customers involves fulfilling orders more accurately and speedily in the short run and managing orders better in the long run. It also requires companies to be responsive to special customer needs and to provide personalized service and continuously increasing value to customers over time.

Implicit in the concept of relationship marketing is the idea of customer selectivity, i.e., that it is not feasible nor worthwhile to establish such relationships with all customers. By focusing resources against those customers who can be profitably served, companies can increase marketing productivity. The profitability of serving different customers is analyzed using "customer retention economics." For example, data from the banking industry indicates that a customer who has been with a bank for five years is several times more profitable than one who has been with the bank for one year. Likewise, it has been estimated that automobile insurance policies have to be held five years before they turn profitable.

Encouraging customer retention and longevity is now recognized as a critical objective in numerous industries, and a variety of "frequent buyer" programs are now offered. While these programs are generally quite cost-effective, their effectiveness is a function of their uniqueness and the value they provide to customers. A company's best customers rightly expect a higher level of customer service and some recognition of their value to the company. Thus, resources can and should be shifted away from other customers to more frequent and loyal customers.

Marketing expenditure for a given customer should decline over time. If not, then those expenditures are being misdirected. However, companies should be careful to allocate an appropriate amount to customer retention, since these customers will drive profitability. Further, the nature of spending has to change over time; the marketing dollars devoted to a client should shift away from advertising and sales promotion to consultative selling, customer business development, and logistical enhancements. Such resources could visibly accumulate in a Customer Business Development fund, and firms should let customers influence how those resources are spent.

Marketing Alliances

In addition to vertical alliances such as those implied by partnering and relationship marketing, companies can also improve their marketing productivity by entering into marketing alliances with other companies. By combining forces with another company interested in reaching a similar target market with a distinct or complementary offering, companies can almost double the productivity of some of their marketing resources. Marketing alliances may most readily be formed for advertising, selling, or distribution. They could also extend into product development or creative product-bundling arrangements.

Another form of marketing alliance is used in "affinity-group" marketing. In such arrangements, companies can market to a group of customers who are members of an affinity group, typically by developing offerings customized for the needs of that group. Their marketing efforts can often piggyback on the communication efforts of the affinity group.

A third type of marketing alliance is one formed in order to engage in "cross-selling." Typically, such alliances are formed between units or divisions of the same company, which may have separate offerings that have appeal to each other's customers. For example, the credit card division of American Express works with the travel and publishing divisions of that company to cross-sell their offerings. Different divisions of a bank may sell diverse services to the same customer. Such capabilities are enhanced through the utilization of Customer Information Files shared across business units. These are an example of data-based marketing, which we discuss later.

Marketing alliances clearly improve marketing efficiency, since they achieve synergy in resource utilization. They also improve marketing effectiveness, since customers are offered convenient "one-stop-shop" access to more products.

Better Domain Definition

An underexplored area in the search for greater marketing productivity is that of defining where marketing tasks should be performed. We have broken this down into two: up the value chain (outsourcing to suppliers) and down the value chain (getting customers to take over some tasks). Used appropriately, both of these approaches achieve effective efficiency, since they lower costs while improving quality and customer satisfaction. A third possibility is to move marketing tasks into other parts of the company that can achieve the same results more efficiently or effectively (or both). For example, certain tasks performed by customer service could be designed into the product, thus reducing the need for customer service.

Make vs. Buy: Insourcing vs. Outsourcing

Some marketing activities, such as advertising, have traditionally been outsourced, and others, such as market research, are increasingly being outsourced. We believe that the marketing function needs to make more informed evaluations of which tasks should be outsourced and which should be brought in-house. Many companies simply do too many activities in-house, while others outsource activities that are very important to retain control over. For example, many firms can profitably outsource relationship creation (through the use of third-party distribution channels, for example), but most firms should *not* outsource relationship management.

Some marketing activities that are candidates for outsourcing include sales, sales management (just as many companies are already outsourcing the human resource function), sales promotion, logistics, marketing information systems, customer service, and so on. Indeed, almost any marketing activity must be evaluated in terms of a "make vs. buy" decision.

If done properly, outsourcing can contribute tremendously to marketing productivity. The reason for this is very simple: outsourcing typically involves taking a secondary or "back-burner" activity and handling it over to a specialist, for whom it is a "front-burner" activity. The specialist enjoys economies of scale and scope in performing the activity; it also provides leading-edge capabilities and can cost-justify investments in emerging technologies. For example, Laura Ashley successfully outsourced its inbound and outbound logistics functions to Federal Express' Business Logistics Division. The result was a 10 percent reduction in costs, coupled with a dramatic improvement in product availability and the launch of a new worldwide, 48-hour direct delivery service.

Getting Customers to Do More Work

One of the ironies of marketing is that customers are often more satisfied when they are themselves able to perform some tasks that marketers would normally perform. Companies could simultaneously lower their costs and increase customer satisfaction by identifying such areas. For example, the leading telecommunications companies have accomplished this by providing billing information to their business customers in a variety of computer media, such as floppy discs, CD-ROMs, and computer tapes. Customers then use software (also provided by the telecommunications company) to analyze the data themselves, rather than have the telecommunications company provide detailed reports.

Often, such opportunities are made possible by allowing customers direct access to company databases. Companies can increase customer satisfaction as well as lower their own costs, since they need not employ personnel to answer certain customer queries. For example, the use of direct dialing for calling cards reduced costs for phone companies and made their customers happier. FedEx, UPS, most of the airlines, and a number of banks are currently using this technology.

Companies can also leverage their own satisfied customers as salespeople. This can either be done explicitly, as MCI has done with its highly successful Friends & Family program, or indirectly, through greater use of "word-of-mouth" marketing. Such approaches have proved to be highly cost effective.

Unbundling and Rebundling Services

Since customer service is rightly viewed as an essential component of good marketing, many firms have become trapped in an escalating spiral of increasing service costs. When such service is bundled along with the core product, it can rapidly increase the costs of marketing and erode profitability. It also leads to the cross-subsidization of one group (heavy users of service) by another (light users). Such hidden cross-subsidization contributes to marketing inefficiency and provides opportunities for competitors to target profitable (i.e., low service) customers by offering them lower prices.

The answer is not to reduce or eliminate service but to unbundle it. By doing so, firms can provide a base level of service to all customers and then offer different levels of service to different customer groups for a fee. Alternatively, it can choose to continue to offer the service for no additional charge to its most frequent and profitable customers. Such an approach increases marketing productivity by increasing revenues (through the sale of value-added services to high-end customers) and lowering costs (by reducing the incidence of unprofitable service provision to other customers). The personal computer software industry has been particularly successful in effecting this transition. Manufacturers offer varying levels of support under different fee structures for different segments of consumers and businesses.

Rationalizing the Marketing Mix

As suggested at the outset of this section, the productivity problem in marketing is often due to resource allocation among the elements of the marketing mix. Productivity can sometimes be improved simpy by pulling back in some areas of marketing spending and deploying all or some part of those resources elsewhere. For example, Procter & Gamble recently cut their spending on sales promotion drastically and increased spending on advertising and R&D.

As mentioned earlier, competitive pressures have led marketers to add more and more variations in elements of the marketing mix. Since these are often unrelated to actual differences in customer preferences, they can add complexity and cost without adding offsetting value. For example, the airline and long-distance industries have proliferated pricing schemes to such a degree that customers are confused and often resentful. We discuss three options for rationalizing the marketing mix below.[12]

Umbrella Branding

While "brand equity" is a powerful force in consumer decision making, it can be very expensive to create and sustain. Companies can often achieve the benefits of a powerful brand name without investing in the resources to create a new name by utilizing brand names where feasible. Of course, this can only be done if the same image is appropriate for both products. The problem with brand extendibility has been that many brands have been defined (mostly through past advertising) in too narrow a fashion. As a result, they become very product-specific and difficult to extend. On the other hand, some firms have been slow to recognize the value of the brand equity in some of their products and have underutilized those assets. For example, Procter & Gamble discovered some years ago that Ivory was really an umbrella brand, not just one that stood for soap. Japanese companies such as Matsushita (Panasonic), Mitsubishi, and Yamaha have been very successful at using their brand names across an extremely wide variety of products.

Rationalizing and Recycling Advertising

Marketers have often struggled with the issue of advertising wearout and have often made two kinds of mistakes: sticking with poor advertising campaigns long after it becomes evident that they are failing; and prematurely terminating very successful campaigns. Both contribute to the problem of marketing productivity.

Marketing productivity in this area has been hurt by the traditional practice of compensating advertising agencies on the basis of a negotiated percentage of media billings. This method creates a perverse incentive for the advertising agency: an outstanding commercial, research has shown, is many times more effective than an average one. However, it needs to be run much less frequently and thus results in lower compensation for the agency. Clearly, in order for the productivity of advertising spending to increase, agencies must be compensated for the effectiveness of their advertising. Further, they must be given incentives to achieve effective results with the lowest possible expenditure on media. This problem is very similar to the conflict of interest that is said to exist between securities brokerages and their clients.

One possible solution is to completely unbundle the creation of advertising from the media scheduling and purchase, as Coca Cola and some other companies have recently done. This practice may accelerate in the future.

A number of companies have successfully "recycled" old advertising campaigns. Such efforts are often but not always tied in to a nostalgia theme. To allow this to occur more often, agencies should be asked to create advertising that is not time-sensitive and thus will not rapidly become dated. Also, advertising agencies can recycle their own creative work by utilizing approaches that have worked well in one context into another, noncompeting context.

Reducing Product Proliferation

Advances in manufacturing now allow many firms to increase the assortment of products they can produce without increasing unit costs. Such advances have been made possible through the adoption of "flexible manufacturing systems" and various software-driven manufacturing processes.

Ironically, this capability has sometimes contributed to declining marketing productivity. It has allowed firms to expand the range of their product offerings beyond what the market needs. However, it has increased the need for advertising and sales forces, and it has also increased the difficulty of forecasting sales, resulting in more unsold inventory. As a result, the marketing costs for the product line increase substantially, lowering or eliminating profits for the line.

The ability to produce products efficiently does not mean you can sell them efficiently. For example, at the time it sold its housewares business to Black & Decker, General Electric produced 150 different products in 14 product categories, including 14 models of irons. To obtain distribution support for its entire line, the company had to administer a whole range of incentive programs for retailers, including early-buy allowances, full-line forcing programs, and so on. After acquiring the business, Black & Decker has gradually moved away from this approach. Instead, the company offers a rationalized product line and relies on a replenishment logistics approach to move toward its stated philosophy of "Sell one, ship one, build one."

Use of Information Technology

Many of the productivity improvements in other aspects of business has been due to the deployment of information technology. Several of the productivity enhancers discussed in the previous section are based upon the use of the new capabilities of today's computing and communications technologies.

We believe that the impact of information technology on marketing has only begun to be felt. In the past decade, scanner systems have enabled marketers in the consumer packaged goods industry to make better-informed and more timely decisions. However, much of what they have done has not changed appreciably. The availability, affordability, and capability of information technology are fast approaching a level where wholesale changes can be considered. Such changes offer the promise of raising marketing productivity to a new level.

The primary technological drivers are the following:

- Greater computing power in ever-smaller form factors at increasingly affordable prices;

- Greater communication bandwidth, along with more availability of wireless data transmission capabilities;

- Increasingly sophisticated and user-friendly software, including the popularization of embedded and stand-alone expert systems;

- Real time capture and distribution of pertinent marketing data, including transaction data as well as various stimulus variables such as advertising; and

- Rapid progress in the area of voice recognition technology.

The impact of these enormously powerful technologies on marketing will be profound. In order to gain their full benefits, it will not be sufficient for marketing to automate and otherwise improve existing ways of doing things. Rather, many marketing processes will have to be *reengineered,* i.e., redesigned "from the ground up" to take advantage of available information tools.

We would like to highlight three factors related to information technology and marketing—the use of data-based marketing and "front-line information systems" and the likely impact of the so-called "information highway" on marketing productivity.

Data-Based Marketing

More and better information about customers is at the heart of marketing. The use of data-based marketing is already fairly advanced, so we will not discuss its fundamentals here. Data-based marketing clearly contributes to greater marketing efficiency through, for example, better targeting of prospects for products and promotions, greater customizability of marketing messages and programs, and so on.

We offer the following observations about the path of data-based marketing in the future:

- Privacy issues will increasingly come to the fore. Unless the marketing profession (not just the Direct Marketing Association) develops an approach to deal with this, it could lead to the imposition of very restrictive rules on the use of customer information. Such rules have already been adopted in Europe.

- Data-based marketing must focus on greater value creation for the customer in addition to marketing efficiency enhancement.

- As technological capabilities expand, all companies will have access to unlimited data and broadband interactive multimedia communication channels with their customers. The difference will be in which companies are best able to use these efficiency-increasing capabilities to best satisfy customers.

Front-Line Information Systems

In the traditional hierarchical corporation, customer contact personnel occupy the lowest tier in terms of status, responsibility, and compensation. However, their impact on customer satisfaction is arguably greater than that of any other group. Typically, in such corporations, the most sophisticated information technology is deployed at the top tier of management for "Executive Information Systems" (EIS). The next priority has tended to be "Management Information Systems" (MIS) for middle managers. Employees below that level have traditionally been provided low-level transaction-support technologies.

This represents a misplaced sense of priorities. The most powerful impact of this technology is felt when it is harnessed at the front-lines, and companies that invest in and deploy cutting-edge front-line information systems (FIS) achieve breakthrough improvements in service quality and reliability, and thus very high levels of consumer satisfaction. Examples include FedEx, Frito Lay and Hertz, each of which equips its front-line personnel with technologies that enable them to do their work faster and better. Not incidentally, such companies also tend to have high levels of employee satisfaction. Further, since they are using sophisticated tools to perform the work, they have already gathered all the data they need for managerial control purposes; such data then "trickle up" into the MIS and EIS levels.

Many companies have already achieved major productivity gains in front-line areas such as sales and customer service. For example, companies that have made sophisticated use of laptop computers and wireless communications for their sales forces have improved their performance and productivity in the areas of account management, lead management, literature fulfillment, reporting (using templates), proposal generation, responding to customer inquiries, quote status, inventory checking, and so on. Anderson Consulting now equips its consultants with a CD-ROM called the "Global Best Practices Knowledge Base," which contain best practice information on about 170 business processes. AT&T, Compaq, and many others now utilize the concept of "hoteling," whereby permanent office space for salespeople is replaced by temporary space on an as-needed basis to encourage salespeople to spend as much time in customer contact as possible.

The priority use of sophisticated FIS, we strongly believe, can lead firms to achieve quantum improvements in the effective efficiency of their marketing activities.

Marketing and the Global Information Highway

The most significant driver of dramatic change in marketing processes in coming years will be the advent of the "information highway." Universal, interactive broadband communication will allow companies to integrate advertising, sales promotion, personal selling, and even distribution to a far greater extent than now possible. It may spell the end of time and place constraints on customers. This technology is likely to become widespread in the U.S. by the year 2005 and will dramatically transform the marketing functions of advertising, personal selling, and physical distribution. It will radically reconfigure industries such as retailing, healthcare, and education, while dramatically affecting nearly all others.

Marketing in this new environment will have to be predicated upon "monocasting" or "pointcasting" of communications, mass customization of all marketing mix elements, a high degree of customer involvement and control, and greater integration between marketing and operations. Companies that are successful in making the transition to this new way of marketing will be characterized by fewer wasted marketing resources and minimal customer alienation resulting from misapplied marketing stimuli. All companies will experience enormous pressures to deliver greater value, more global competition, and intense jostling for the loyalties of "desirable" customers.

Better Monitoring and Control

Tracking, monitoring, directing activity—they are the essence of management. New techniques and technologies will make these functions more effective and efficiency-enhancing.

Adjusting Compensation of Marketing Personnel

In order to improve effective efficiency, companies must create transparent incentive schemes that focus all marketing personnel on the essentials: increasing the profitability of what they do and simultaneously increasing customer satisfaction. Companies such as IBM have adopted precisely those two criteria in determining salesforce compensation. Such approaches could be spread into all areas of marketing.

An important related issue is the compensation of advertising agencies, which was discussed earlier under "Rationalizing and Recycling Advertising."

Continuous Assessment of Marketing Practices

As in any other human or business endeavor, there is substantial inertia in marketing practices. In other words, new practices are added on slowly, and old ones are discarded even more slowly. As with creeping product proliferation, marketing programs have a way of accumulating by perpetuating themselves even after they have outlived their usefulness.

Michael Treacy has suggested that innovative marketing programs start to lose their effectiveness after three or four companies adopt them.[13] It is important to distinguish here between short-lived marketing innovations and those that represent a lasting improvement. The latter may cease to be sources of competitive advantage after others adopt them, but are certainly not candidates for termination. We believe that the relationship marketing paradigm falls under this category.

Marketers could achieve addition through subtraction by periodically reviewing and rationalizing the whole gamut of marketing activities, programs, and offerings. As always, the criteria to use, we believe, should be whether or not the elements in question contribute to the achievement of effective efficiency.

Some Cautions in Seeking Productivity Improvements

While we have attempted to show numerous ways in which the marketing function can become more productive, some words of caution are in order. It can readily be discerned that marketing's track record in the use of efficiency tools has not been a stellar one. Tools such as telemarketing and database marketing have often been applied in a manner that has increased customer alienation. Companies have focused on efficiency to the near-exclusion of effectiveness. In Ted Levitt's terminology, they have focused on the needs of the seller rather than the buyer.

While our definition of marketing productivity, if adopted, should prevent such abuses, we would like to reiterate that message here. Too much short-term productivity pressure may increase what we term the "malpractices of marketing," practices such as deceptive advertising and selling, price gouging and so on.

Another danger is that an intense push for marketing productivity could lead to an exodus of talented people from the organization. An excessive focus on short-term productivity measures could lead to a reduction in the types of marketing expenditures which are rightly viewed as long-term investments.[14]

Conclusion

The push for productivity in marketing spending is in no way contradictory to creating and maintaining a market orientation. Being customer-oriented does not necessarily mean having to spend more on marketing. The fact is that too many companies use marketing dollars as a blunt weapon. They seem to believe that if they spend enough they will become customer-oriented. Thus they subject the customer to a barrage of redundant advertising and numerous sales promotions. To a customer who has already bought the company's product, much of this is wasted spending; in fact, that customer is subsidizing the profligate and poorly focused spending of the company. Focused and tailored marketing spending is not only more efficient, it also reduces the amount of marketing noise and improves customer contentment.

Marketing reform must come from within, rather than be imposed from above. That is the only way to ensure that the changes that result increase the efficiency as well as the effectiveness of marketing actions. This concept of "effective efficiency" guides all of the recommendations we have put forward. Marketing in the future will be called upon to make an even greater contribution to the corporation than it has in the past. More and more, corporate "top line" success (i.e., revenues and market share) will depend on the quality of their marketing efforts. At the same time, corporate "bottom-line" success (i.e., profitability) will depend on how cost-effectively marketing is able to perform its tasks.

Notes

1. Michael P. Sullivan (1991), "CEOs Are Asking about Declining Productivity in Marketing," *The American Banker,* January 7, 1991, pg. 4.

2. Sullivan, op. cit.

3. John M. Berry, "For Many Firms, Benefit of Cutting Inventories Is Worth the Risk," *The Washington Post,* October 6, 1994, product. D1.

4. Matt Walsh, "Point of Sale Persuaders," *Forbes,* October 24, 1994, pg. 232–234.

5. Nil Houston (1948), *Methods of Efficiency Analysis in Marketing,* Harvard University Ph.D. Dissertation, pg. 344; cited in Buzzell (below).

6. Robert D. Buzzell (1957), *Marketing Productivity,* Ohio State University, Ph.D. Dissertation.

7. Philip Kotler, *Marketing Management,* 8th Edition, Prentice-Hall, 1994.

8. For example, see Thomas A. Steward, "Your Company's Most Valuable Asset: Intellectual Capital," *Fortune,* October 3, 1994, pg. 68–74.

9. For an excellent description of ABC and its role in marketing, see Robin Cooper and Robert S. Kaplan, "Measure Costs Right: Make the Right Decisions," *Harvard Business Review,* September-October 1988.

10. *Quick Response News,* December 9, 1991.

11. *Efficient Consumer Response: Enhancing Consumer Value in the Grocery Industry,* Kurt Salmon Associates, Inc., January 1993.

12. The term "rationalizing" in this connection has been used by Fred Wiersema of the CSC/Index Consulting Group. See CSC Index Alliance presentations on *Lean Marketing: The Immediate Imperative* by Fred Wiersema ("More Bang for the Buck") and Michael Treacy ("The Strategic Context for Lean Marketing") at the Executive Forum, Tucson, Arizona, December 1993.

13. Michael Treacy, op. cit.

14. See, for example, Adrian J. Slywotzky and Benson P. Shapiro, "Leveraging to Beat the Odds: The New Marketing Mind-Set," *Harvard Business Review,* September-October 1993, pg. 97–107.

Section VI
Micromarkets and Micromarketing

Many of the articles in this book have either had as their subject or at least alluded to the death of the mass market and the rise of smaller and smaller special markets. This section explores the special marketing acumen needed to sell to these new and increasingly important constituencies.

In "Tapping the Mature Market" Robert Menchin defines and explains the ten trends related to the "graying of America" that will make the over-65 market the most lucrative one for marketers who know how to tap its strength. In "The Moving Target: A Guide to Reaching the Women's Market," Rena Bartos dissects traditional explanations and definitions of marketing to women and explains the shortcomings of those approaches. In particular, she describes how there isn't a single market but rather many markets defined by different needs driven by a host of factors, some easily understood, others much more complex.

There is an inescapable irony in the fact that, on one hand, so much of the change in marketing has been driven by technology and, on the other hand, that technology marketing itself has been so miserable. So says Kate Bertrand in "Technology Marketing Grows Up," as she predicts a new day in marketing technology-related products in which the shoemaker's children will no longer go barefoot. In a very different growth area, "Sports Marketing," Howard Schlossberg describes some of the forces driving sports marketing and analyzes the increasing sophistication that will characterize this dynamic area.

In yet another specialty area, the travel industry, Barry Smith explains how "Yield Management" will help successful travel-oriented businesses of the future cope with the special vicissitudes of their industry. In the next article, "Electric Utility Marketing," Jerry Neal describes the marketing initiatives that these near-monopolies of the past must take to survive and prosper in the future. And in "The Changing Seasons of Marketing," Judith Waldrop surveys the many marketing opportunities afforded by events and celebrations connected with special holidays observed by the growing number of ethnic groups in the United States.

—36—
TAPPING THE
MATURE MARKET

Robert S. Menchin

Robert S. Menchin is a recognized authority on marketing to mature consumers. In a career spanning more than 25 years, he has written four books and hundreds of articles, brochures, booklets, ads, direct mail campaigns, newsletters, sales presentations, and seminar programs for Fortune 500 companies and other major international firms. As former Vice President of Member Relations and Communications of the Chicago Board of Trade (the oldest and largest futures exchange in the world) and head of Wall Street Marketing Communications (a Chicago-based consulting firm), he has an established following in the mature marketing network.

When the jail psychologist asked the legendary Willie Sutton why he robbed banks, he answered, "That's where the money is." For the thousands of successful businesses catering to the mature market, it's as simple as that. That's where the money is. The 62 million people age 50 and over (one of every four people in the United States) represent a huge and profitable market for goods and services (see Table 1). They have a combined annual income of more than $160 billion in discretionary income.

Futurescope

Catering to the needs and desires of America's older population is a growth industry as we approach the year 2000. Ten major trends make that statement a reality:

1. The more than 60 million Americans 50 and over represent a larger number of seniors than ever before in history.

2. The senior population represents an increasingly larger proportion of the total U.S. population.

3. As a group, today's seniors are healthier and more active than previous generations of older Americans.

4. With dramatic increases in life expectancy, the current older population will have many more years of life.

5. Today's seniors have a more positive self-image and a more active life-style.

6. Today's seniors are more financially secure and have more disposable income than any other population segment.

7. The trend toward earlier retirement gives seniors more years of free time and leisure.

8. There are many more women than men in the older segment of the population.

9. As the total U.S. population becomes older, society's attitude toward older men and women and personal perceptions of aging have become more positive.

10. Even greater growth in the number and changes in the character of the older generation lie ahead as the oldest baby boomers become seniors.

Table 1   Number of Americans in Various Age Segments
(Total U.S. population, 243.9 million)

	Million	**Percent**
50 and over	62.7	25.7
55 and over	51.8	21.3
65 and over	29.8	12.3
70 and over	19.9	8.2
80 and over	6.3	2.6
50 to 54	10.9	4.5
55 to 64	22.0	9.0
65 to 79	9.8	4.1
70 to 74	7.7	3.2
75 to 79	5.7	2.4

Catering to the needs and desires of this burgeoning mature market is a great growth industry of the future. Our current generation of seniors lives longer, healthier, and more financially secure lives than any previous generation of older Americans. Their physical and mental health is better than any generation of seniors that came before. Today's more active, bigger-spending senior population is a prime target for every kind of goods and services. And not just for over-the-counter medicines and retirement housing, the products usually associated with older men and women. Mature people are top prospects for goods and services not usually associated with the later years. They buy exercise equipment, running shoes, household appliances, cruise vacations, and the better automobiles.

Keys to Mature Market Success

There are three keys to success in the mature market:

1. Produce goods and services that fill the special needs of seniors.

2. Shape your marketing strategy and your advertising message to attract the older consumer.

3. Media must be researched carefully to find the most efficient and cost-effective way of reaching your prospects.

Table 2   Acronyms for Key Segments of the Mature Market

WHOPPIES:	Well-Heeled Older People
OPALS:	Older Persons with Active Life-Styles
GRUMPIES:	Grown Up Mature People
ACES:	Active, College-Educated Seniors
SUPPIES:	Senior Urban Professionals

Let's explore each of these keys to mature market success.

Producing Goods and Services to Fill Specific Needs

Although as marketing professionals you might have little input in designing what you sell, you should know that the companies that are most successful in selling to seniors are those that bring marketing into the process.

When book sales representatives told the book publishers that their older customers pass up worthy books because the type is too small and gravitate to books with larger, more readable text, the large-type book was born. Today, whole new sections of bookstores and mail-order book clubs are devoted to large-type editions of books: classics, popular novels, and even bibles are now among the best-selling books.

In the insurance business, new insurance products have been designed to cater to the senior policyholder. New health-insurance policies fill the gap between government medical benefits and the total cost of a senior's medical bills. Long-term care insurance was created to keep seniors from going broke if they have to go into a nursing home. The insurance industry has also designed special annuity investment programs for seniors who want to buy guaranteed income for the rest of their lives. Health-insurance policies and annuities are among the best-selling and most profitable insurance products being sold today.

In addition to serving the current senior population, what these industries are really doing is tracking the baby boomer generation. Every 40 seconds another person in the United States turns 50. In 1996 the first of the large post-war generation will reach their 50th birthday. Each year, millions of baby boomers will become seniors, swelling the senior population to numbers even greater than we see today. The mature market is a moving target, and if you want to hold on to your customers you have to relate to their changing needs and preferences as they age (see Table 2).

Shaping Marketing Strategy and Advertising
to Relate to the Needs, Preferences, and Sensibilities
of Older Men and Women

Talk to people in the language of their perceived age, not their chronological age. Research shows that most seniors perceive themselves as being 10–15 years younger than they actually are. So, if you want your ads aimed at mature men and women to be effective, focus on people at least 10–15 years younger.

More than anything else, seniors want substance, not glitter. So use a soft-sell approach and as much copy as it takes to tell the full story. They have the time and patience to read it all and evaluate it carefully. As seasoned shoppers, they want value for their money, and they recognize quality when they see it.

Older consumers are more interested in purchasing "experiences" than they are in purchasing "things." Mature people have filled their homes with things. In their later years, they want products and services that help them enjoy experiences and self-fulfillment.

Special discounts for seniors have become an expected advantage, and older consumers seek out and do business where they have an edge. So, if possible, build in a special advantage that can be labeled "senior discount" or its equivalent. It works like a charm with value-conscious seniors.

Developing the Most Efficient and Cost-Effective
Ways of Reaching Senior Customers

Do you market children's toys? You can buy television time on a Saturday morning children's TV show or take a full-page ad in *Humpty Dumpty* magazine or next to the comics in your local paper. If I were selling toys, I would advertise in a medium that caters to the 50-plus set. Nobody but nobody buys toys as enthusiastically and as generously as grandma and grandpa.

It is interesting to note that NBC, the network that has always programmed to attract the younger audience, is at the bottom of the ratings contest and has been losing ground to the other networks. At the same time, CBS, the television network that specifically targets older viewers, is number one in the ratings and is the most profitable of the major networks. This is a dramatic example of demographics at work.

Television, radio, and print are all effective in reaching seniors. But a recent study by the Roper Organization reveals that mature adults have the most respect for print advertising. They find most of the ads they read in magazines and newspapers to be useful and informative.

Advertisers seeking a cost-effective audience for their message can choose a publication specifically targeted to 50-plus seniors or one with editorial content heavily weighted with content of interest to seniors. Of these, I believe that magazines for seniors are the most effective, because the senior's publication is "the trade journal of the retiree." Just as trade and professional journals are important for business people and professionals, senior publications are must reading for many mature people. My research shows that senior publications—local senior newspapers and national magazines—are read thoroughly and referred to often. Virtually everything in senior publications is pertinent to seniors, and almost 90 percent of the content is not available in any other medium.

Two of the largest-circulation magazines in the United States, *Modern Maturity* and *New Choices,* are specifically for seniors. *Modern Maturity* is the magazine for the 31 million members of the American Association of Retired Persons (AARP), making it the largest-circulation magazine in the United States. *New Choices* magazine, a large-circulation senior magazine, is owned by Reader's Digest. Senior magazines in the United States are popular with advertisers because they deliver the audience and because they are read. The Roper Poll finds that seniors spend several hours each week reading magazines, and a great deal of it is spent with magazines specifically for seniors.

A few mechanical tips on creating ads for older consumers: Use large type. Avoid reverse type for body copy—it's more difficult to read. In your ad layout, color is less important than sharp contrast. Make response convenient. Cut-out coupons should be easy to get at. It should be very clear in your ad how to buy or where to find your product or service. Some of these mechanical tips might seem obvious, but it's amazing how often they are overlooked.

This review of the three keys to selling to the mature market, (1) creating the right product, (2) shaping the message, and (3) using the most cost-efficient media, covers the basics. But the orientation of the marketer to the older consumer is not complete without a thorough understanding of the attitudes and consumer behavior of mature people.

Understanding Mature Consumer Behavior

Seniors in the United States find themselves in a serious financial squeeze. The $900 billion cited earlier is the combined income of our 50-plus population. Individual income is something else. In the United States, most people retire with incomes at about half of the income they had at the prime of their work life. It's no surprise, therefore, that seniors are careful about money. They are determined to get value for each dollar, but at the same time they are willing to spend on themselves and eager to enjoy life.

Many of today's seniors are less concerned with leaving money and property to their children and more interested in enjoying their money now. I noticed a bumper sticker on an automobile that seems to sum it all up: "I'm spending my grandchildren's inheritance."

Career Opportunities

As this century ends and a new century begins, marketers who target older consumers will find the demographics on their side. Marketing professionals seeking to develop their career in a lucrative and dynamic niche would do well to concentrate on this market. Those who do will be part of a growing but select group of marketing people to reap the rewards of this powerful demographic trend. Recently, *Working Woman* magazine listed "marketing for the mature market" as one of the 25 hottest careers. Companies throughout the United States and Europe are keeping an eye out for marketing people with skill and experience in selling to seniors.

The era of a youth-focused consumer market is coming to an end, and it will not be seen again in our lifetimes. In sheer numbers and in spending power, the senior market is a valuable prize to be won by those who relate to the needs and desires of consumers age 55 and over. They are the fastest-growing population segment in the United States, Europe, and the developed nations in the Pacific. In today's aging world, no company can afford to ignore this market.

—37—
THE MOVING TARGET

A Guide to Reaching the Women's Market

Rena Bartos

Rena Bartos is President of the Rena Bartos Company. A consultant and writer, she counsels on communications and consumer issues, and is the author of *Marketing to Women Around the World, The Moving Target: What Every Marketer Should Know About Women, Advertising and Consumers—New Perspectives, The Future of the Advertising Agency Research Function,* and *The Founding Fathers of Advertising Research.* She was formerly a Senior Vice President and Director of Communications Development at the J. Walter Thompson Company. She holds degrees from Rutgers University and Columbia University.

I believe that the women's market is a moving target. To be more precise, it is a number of targets not all moving at the same time and not necessarily going in the same direction. The key to reaching those targets is to link changing demography and changing values to your day-to-day marketing actions. I will spell out some ways that you can create those linkages. There are two stages in the marketing process in which these applications can be most useful: at the beginning or at the end. The first basic step in any marketing program is to define or redefine the target group. It is here that the new demographic realities can have the most impact in identifying new opportunities. At the end of the process, when those opportunities are translated into advertising, an understanding of the changing social values and the changing aspirations of consumers can assure that your marketing communications will achieve maximum credibility and maximum relevance to their intended targets.

I will challenge some of your pet assumptions about consumers and question some of the conventional wisdom that is passed on by one brand manager or department head to another. I find that the greatest obstacle to implementing change lies not in our techniques, but in our underlying assumptions about society, which are rarely examined and never challenged. Many marketers have unexamined assumptions about the market, about consumers, and about advertising. If any of those assumptions are out of sync with reality, all of the technology and sophisticated methodology invested in their models could result in anything from missed opportunities to outright marketing disasters. On a more basic level, unexamined assumptions might be built into the way research is designed. If those assumptions aren't clarified before the questionnaire is written, there is no way to rescue the situation after the fact.

The Quiet Revolution

There is one simple demographic fact that is the basis of a quiet revolution: The dramatic rise in the number of women in the United States who go to work. The

Futurescope

It is clear from current demographic trends that women's economic role in the 21st century will have a profound effect on marketing techniques and goals. Marketers with vision will sweep away their outdated preconceptions of the women's market and embrace new demographic and market-analysis tools that will allow them to reach all segments of this increasingly diverse market segment. Those who refuse to address changing demography and social values will find it impossible to reap the rewards of women's growing financial power.

flood of women entering the work force is not only a major demographic trend, but also the manifestation of a profound social change. Professor Eli Ginzberg, former chairman of the National Commission for Manpower Policy, calls it "the single most outstanding phenomenon of our century." In 1990, 58 percent of all women in the United States 16 years of age and over were in the labor force. But the number of women who work is only part of the story. If 58 percent of all women in our country go to work, we might assume that the remaining 42 percent must be at home keeping house. Actually, only 25 percent of women are full-time homemakers. The remaining are out of the mainstream. They are either still in school or they are retired and/or disabled. Thirty-three percent more women are working out of the house than are staying home and keeping house. Working women really are the majority of all active women in our country. This is a fact that some marketers have not yet absorbed. Once we remove the schoolgirls and the retired grandmothers from the picture, the ratio of working women to housewives is 70 to 30 percent.

Action Implications

The action implications of this fact are also clear, but they are not always followed. Traditionally, many marketing and advertising efforts were aimed at housewives. Therefore, in view of the current realities, it makes sense to compare the consumer needs of full-time homemakers with those of working women. Unfortunately, some marketers simply compare working women to non-working women, without isolating the full-time homemakers from the non-working segment.

Please note that a major piece of research on the women's market suffers from this flaw. While the design carefully codified attitudes and behavior on a great many issues, the only occupational question asked was whether a woman is employed. Therefore, the non-working women in that sample lumps full-time homemakers with schoolgirls and retired women. This means that there is no way to isolate the traditional target group of full-time housewives in the analysis.

The Concept of Life Cycle

Let's assume you have, in fact, separated homemakers from other non-working women. Is that all there is to it? I'm afraid just comparing working women to housewives is painting with too broad a brush. All working women are not alike, nor are all housewives. Neither group is monolithic. What's more, they never were! One clue to their diversity is their position in the life cycle. Are they married or not? Do they have any children at home?

Even though we tend to think of the typical American woman as a wife with 2.4 kiddies holding on to her apron strings, the reality is that only 54 percent of American women are married. So, even if they wanted to, more than four in ten women could not possibly follow the 1950s pattern of shopping for the family while hubby is off at work and the children are at school. Some marketers assume that in the typical American family, the wife stays home and cares for the house and children and the husband goes to work to support the family. However, the reality is that 8 percent of women are married to men who are out of the work force because of retirement or health reasons. Among those with at least one working spouse, there are almost three times as many working wives as women who live in the traditional pattern of breadwinner husband and homemaker wife. The two-paycheck marriage has really become the norm.

Action Implications

This new reality has research implications as well. It doesn't take a rocket scientist to compare the consumer behavior of working wives and non-working wives. In every case, the working wives are better customers. However, many researchers have not related this to the consumer potential of their husbands. Back in the early 1970s, when I first analyzed the market behavior of working and non-working wives, it occurred to me that the simple fact of a wife's working would affect the way that household spends its money. Two men could be identical in education, income, and occupation, but if one was married to a working wife and one to a full-time homemaker, that one simple demographic fact could make them very different consumers. Yet at that time they could not be identified in any marketing study because no one had thought of asking men, "What does your wife do?"

The marketing implications here are to consider the occupation of the spouse in assessing the consumer potential of either men or women. It just requires asking one simple question, but you do have to remember to ask it.

Certainly the consumer needs and life-styles of both working women and housewives are affected by whether they have any young children in their households. Actually, only 34 percent of women in the United States have children under 18 years of age living at home. The majority, some 66 percent, have no kiddies running around the house. When we combine the two demographic facts of marital status and presence of children, we create four life-cycle groups: Married with Children, Childless Married Couples, Not Married/No Children, Single Parents. The traditional vision of the American family as breadwinner husband, homemaker wife, and 2.4 kiddies is so outmoded that some marketers call it the great American myth. Consider this: If we remove the 25 percent of full families from the picture, it becomes clear that 75 percent of American women live in nontraditional life-styles. They are either childless couples, singles, or single parents.

The marketing applications here are very straightforward. You get a much clearer picture of the consumer needs of both working women and housewives if you consider them within the context of their place in the life cycle. Most marketing studies include marital status and presence of children as standard demographic questions. A simple cross-tabulation of these two items creates a life-cycle framework. Past studies of the marketplace can be reanalyzed from this perspective, and of course future studies should build the life-cycle framework in as a matter of course. And remember to identify which men are married to full-time homemakers and which are married to working wives.

The New Demographics

There is another way to sharpen our understanding of both full-time homemakers and working women. I call this approach "the New Demographics." This is a way of segmenting women that divides housewives into those who want to stay at home and those who say they'd like to go to work. We separate working women who think the work they do is "just a job" from those who are career oriented. These four groups of women are very different kinds of people and very different in their potential as consumers. Stay-at-Home Housewives tend to be the oldest and least educated of any group of women in the country. Plan-to-Work Housewives are by far the youngest. They are most likely to have young children. Just-a-Job Working Women begin to get a little younger every year as the plan-to-work housewives really go to work. Career Women are differentiated by education and affluence. They are the best educated. They're most likely to have gone to college or beyond. They are the most affluent of all segments of women.

Action Implications

How can you factor this New Demographic perspective into your marketing strategies? Because these are new questions, not included in your past marketing studies, I urge you to add them to current and future research into the women's market. This does not require a special research project, but rather one additional demographic question for each respondent in any study you might do normally. One question is asked of housewives; another is asked of working women.

Those of you whose companies subscribe to either Simmons Market Research Bureau (SMRB) or Mediamark Research, Inc. (MRI) can have this kind of analysis done tomorrow. Both SMRB and MRI incorporate the New Demographic questions into their databases, so you can analyze the way the New Demographic segments use your product or brand or how they respond to media. The attitudes and values systems of the New Demographic groups can be obtained from the Roper Organization or from the Gallup Poll. Each of these asks the New Demographic questions from time to time. For those of you interested in international marketing, I am happy to tell you that the questions are incorporated in ongoing market and media-tracking studies in the United Kingdom, in Germany, and in Japan.

By expanding your analysis of housewives and working women within the life cycle to include the New Demographics as well, you create a 16-cell analytic model, which combines the four life cycle and the four New Demographic groups. This framework will enable you to evaluate the market potential of the New Demographic and life cycle segments. An objective appraisal of their marketing behavior can tell whether they buy or use products differently or whether their media behavior is distinctive. an equally objective appraisal of their incidence or volume of product use can identify the potential each group represents for a product category or brand. Reanalysis of existing data and of the information available in some of the standard databases like MRI and SMRB will enable you to know the size of each group, exactly which products and brands it buys and how much, and how to reach them through media. Therefore, the results are actionable.

Changing Social Values

So far, all of the applications I have discussed impact on how you define your target group and pinpoint the marketing strategies most relevant to their needs. Let's assume you have done your homework and come out the other end with a finely honed strategy. Now the challenge is to turn it into communications that will motivate those potential targets. Just as changing demography can help you define your target group more sharply, their changing social values mean that you can't talk to them as though we were back in the 1950s. I believe that the surge of women into the work force is only one manifestation of more profound social change. The changing role of women reflects a fundamental change in how women feel about themselves. They have gone beyond derived status, that is, being defined as somebody's daughter, somebody's wife, or somebody's mother. Even the most devoted wife and mother wants to feel like someone in her own right. When Sally Ride took off into space, she really changed the context of the discussion about women. When reporters asked her how it felt to be the first woman in space, she answered that she didn't know what all the fuss was about. She went on to wonder why it took them so long to make the space program accessible to women. She has become the symbol of what women can achieve when they are given access to opportunity.

Action Implications

I suggest that you build the perspective of those target consumers into your creative research and developmental advertising research. I know this is Marketing 101, but you can avoid a lot of grief if you not only identify your potential customers, but also talk to them in order to understand their hopes and dreams as well as their wants and needs in relation to your product. Listening to your target consumers at an early stage in the creative process will enable you to understand the nuances of their self-perceptions and avoid inappropriate stereotypes or alienating executions. I suggest that you use the New Demographic questions as screening questions for any qualitative studies you do of the attitudes of your target consumers or the way they respond to advertising.

How Do You Define Advertising Effectiveness?

Most of the growing skepticism and challenge to advertising comes from our very best customers. Baby boomers are the best-educated generation in our history. Career-oriented working women are apt to be college educated, or better. They are also the most sophisticated and skeptical consumers. They challenge authority figures and conventional wisdom. We see examples of this in the gender gap in how women vote and in growing distrust of politicians and business institutions. Until very recently, the conventional wisdom was that if consumers enjoy the advertising they see, it might be too soft to break through the competitive clutter. As a matter of fact, some practitioners thought that a certain amount of irritation is necessary to achieve effectiveness. The dimension of like and dislike is not usually measured in conventional copy tests. Most practitioners either don't measure it at all or ignore it if it surfaces in their findings. There seems to be an unspoken assumption that "If we don't measure it, it doesn't exist." At best, they consider it a diagnostic measure.

The Advertising Research Foundation recently reported on a study that validates a variety of copy-testing methods against actual sales results. This breakthrough study was over a dozen years in the making. Its objective was "to determine the predictive validity of copy research." One of its specific objectives was to answer the question, "Which individual measures do the best job?" More than 30 individual copy-testing measures were subjected to a rigorous controlled experiment. The criterion used was whether the measure predicted sales results at a statistically significant level. When the author of the report presented the results, he said, "Now brace yourself for a surprise!" The surprise was that the like/dislike scale performed better than any other test measure in predicting sales results. The measure that the pundits had dismissed as too soft was actually the best predictor of effectiveness.

Action Implications

My next suggestion is a more radical one. I suggest that you expand your current copy-testing system to include some measures of emotional response. If you limit your decision-making process to narrow definitions of advertising effectiveness, you might be communicating the right copy points in the wrong tone of voice, and that tonality could boomerang by alienating the very consumers you want to reach. Therefore, I urge you to add some measure of emotional response to your ongoing copy-testing procedures. I believe that it will help you to produce advertising that is effective and that at the same time will enhance the quality of your brand's image and will not undermine its credibility.

I've tried to suggest some very specific ways you can build the changing demography and changing social values of the women's market into your day-to-day marketing activities. I know it is uncomfortable to trod an uncharted path, but the rewards can be great. A long time ago, a duck-hunting friend of mine told me that the way to hit a moving target is to aim at where it is going to be, not at where it's been!

–38–
TECHNOLOGY MARKETING GROWS UP

Kate Bertrand

Kate Bertrand is a freelance writer based in Pacifica, California. Former editor of *Software Marketing Journal* and former West Coast editor of *Business Marketing*, Ms. Bertrand has written for *Advertising Age, Marketing Computers, British Business,* and many other business and consumer publications. She co-authored *Developing a Winning JIT Marketing Strategy* with Charles O'Neal, and has contributed to textbooks on marketing, advertising, and biology.

Forward movement in a product's life cycle inevitably reshapes every aspect of marketing that product, as the maturation of the microcomputer hardware and software market so aptly illustrates.

When microcomputer systems first came on the market in the early 1980s, technological features provided the main difference between models. Computer speed and power, not promotion and pricing, differentiated the various models and drove sales. Although microtechnology has continued to evolve since then at an astonishingly rapid rate, market changes have displaced technology from its role as the most important component of systems selling and made marketing the key to competitive success.

The rapid growth of companies selling hardware and/or software, teamed with a higher level of computer literacy among both business buyers and consumers, has forced vendors to learn about and execute pricing, promotion, product differentiation, and positioning strategies. Distribution also has changed as buyers have become comfortable buying computer systems without the intensive, protracted hand-holding required in the early 1980s.

The influx of competition in hardware and software markets in the past decade has transformed these products into commodities, chipping away at many vendors' earnings and market share and forcing numerous companies out of business. The firms positioned for survival have developed marketing strategies responsive to the reshaped market, with an emphasis on value—high performance at a low price—and ease of purchasing. This is particularly true among hardware marketers.

Formerly premium-priced market leaders such as IBM, Compaq, and Apple, stinging from low-priced mail-order and foreign competition, have introduced systems that offer plenty of speed and power at rock-bottom prices. They have put their faith in this approach's ability to stem share erosion, while acknowledging the margin squeeze it creates.

The pricing shift has teamed up with another important trend, enhanced computer literacy, to reshape microcomputer distribution. Specifically, direct market-

Futurescope

As computer hardware and software marketing enters the new century, increased promotional expenditures on consumer-style promotion, including contests, couponing, rebates, and sampling, seems assured. At the same time, more aggressive product, pricing, and distribution stategies will emerge to meet the changing needs of the maturing microcomputer market. The only marketing constant will be change.

ing and mass merchandising have become the channels of choice for business buyers as well as consumers. Hardware and software vendors are deploying a much broader range of direct-marketing tools than even a few years ago. Favored vehicles include catalogs, call-to-action print ads and advertorials, telemarketing and database marketing programs, and direct-mail campaigns. Meanwhile, superstores and computer warehouses are doing land-office business as savvy hardware buyers shop for high-value products.

To support the more mature approaches to product marketing, pricing, and distribution, leading hardware and software vendors have adopted the kind of aggressive branding strategies commonplace in package-goods marketing but seldom used for business-to-business technology marketing. Some chip manufacturers are even moving in this direction. Intel, for example, is creating awareness for its microprocessor brand with a co-op ad program that has splashed the Intel name over thousands of pages of OEM print ads.

Moreover, advertising media commonly associated with consumer goods, such as television and outdoor, are taking on a new role in the media strategies of a growing number of hardware and software vendors. Expanding on the traditional business-to-business TV approach of buying time during news and sports programming, Intel, WordPerfect, CompuAdd, Microsoft, and a few others have made prime-time and/or cable programming key components in their TV ad schedules. Meanwhile, companies such as IBM, laptop maker Toshiba, and software marketer Corel are building awareness with billboards in major metropolitan markets.

—39—
SPORTS MARKETING

Howard Schlossberg

Howard Schlossberg is the author of a forthcoming book on sports marketing for Blackwell Publishers. He wrote a column on sports marketing for three years in the American Marketing Association's biweekly magazine, *Marketing News.* For the past 20 years, Schlossberg has covered prep athletics in the Chicago area, first for Pioneer Press and currently for Paddock Publications. His coverage has been recognized for excellence by the Northern Illinois Newspaper Association, the Suburban Newspaper of America, and the National Association of Softball Writers and Broadcasters. He also contributes to the hockey magazine *Blueline,* and is Chicago correspondent for the Sports Network wire service. He teaches journalism at William Rainey Harper College.

Just what is it that drives the sports fan to the point of emotional frenzy for the sake of close association with his or her heroes? Those marketers who can properly answer that question, or come as close as possible to doing so, are the ones who are best leveraging sports marketing opportunities. For them, sports marketing—or, more appropriately, marketing through sports—has become an integrated facet of the overall marketing plan, a vehicle for successfully targeting and reaching best customers, and an instrument producing increasingly measurable results.

Advances in Assessing Effectiveness

The marketing research world is approaching the same sophistication in measuring the benefits of sports marketing as its clients are in achieving execution of it, whether it be through an NBA arena, a soccer stadium, a community park district softball league, or a local grade school fitness/nutrition training program. GRPs, CPMs, and Nielsen ratings are no longer the only guidance system or judgment devices. Sports certainly have mass appeal, but savvy sports marketers identify the target audience within the masses with which to associate their product or service.

This is why Volvo sponsors men's professional tennis in addition to grass-roots activities like leagues and clinics at tennis clubs. It's why McDonald's is in everything from high schools to high-flying slam dunks. It's why Michael Jordan wears Nikes. It's why auto-racing telecasts on ESPN on Sunday afternoons approach ratings equal to simultaneously broadcast NFL regional games on the major networks.

Futurescope

Increasingly sophisticated sports marketing research of the 21st century will be able to determine who watched an athletic event (on TV or in person) and why, as well as what the equivalent media exposure would have been for the event sponsor who chose instead to pay out big bucks to networks for advertising time. Decisions on where to direct media and promotional dollars will increasingly be driven by this sophistication in identifying audience appeal, as marketers see the value in the efficiencies of sponsorship over mass media in cost, targeting, and ultimately in successful marketing strategies. As more effective technologies drive more efficient global marketing, corporate marketers and event sponsors and owners will become the kinds of marketing partners that ad agencies like to think they are with their clients.

It's why you see packaged-goods logos you would never expect on race cars (more than 40 percent of some auto-racing audiences are female).

It's why households across America shell out the bucks for pay-per-view telecasts of championship boxing matches and showdown wrestling clashes, but stay away in droves from even the most deeply discounted Olympic TripleCast pay-per-view offerings. The events and their performers, in and of themselves, are the promotional vehicles. They create their own value levels with consumers (also known as fans).

The Mysterious Power of Sports Marketing

Why do fans seemingly sell their souls to be close to the sports—and athletes—they develop adoration for? Why do pay-per-view packages work for some events and sports, and not others? Who is willing to test the waters—and the corporate bank account—to find out? Apparently, many are. Boxing and wrestling remain pay-per-view hits, but mainstream sports like football and basketball can't make significant inroads, because fans won't let them. They have clearly told marketers where to draw the line.

Sports marketing—mainly sponsorship—is flying high in sophistication and growing in popularity in the range of billions of dollars. However, it is also facing tremendously difficult decisions that will leave sponsoring bodies, sports moguls, corporate sponsors, and especially fans with increasingly difficult choices.

How to leverage sports marketing opportunities and still develop a better handle on what make Joe Consumer tick will drive tighter relationships between all sports marketing parties, ensuring their drive toward mutually beneficial results. Heightening competition in an increasingly cluttered entertainment marketplace (and that's just on the TV screen) will surely drive more sophisticated and integrated marketing programs by operators on all sides of the sports marketing relationship to ensure measurable results, profitability, sales, awareness, exposure, and goodwill benefits.

In the meantime, did you hear the one about the guy who told his wife to put the gourmet snack food back on the shelf at the grocery store and to buy generic snacks instead—just before he forked over a few hundred dollars to scalpers for football playoff tickets?

That's why sponsorship is a more than $3-billion-a-year business, and licensed sports merchandise accounts for nearly 20 percent of all licensed merchandise sold in the United States. Pro baseball, football, and basketball alone each record more than $1 billion a year in licensed merchandise sales. You and I are the reasons why. And we always will be as long as there's a Shaquille O'Neal, Michael Jordan, Joe Montana, Wayne Gretzky, or Roger Clemens out there for us to worship.

—40—
YIELD MANAGEMENT
A Strategic Tool for the Travel Industry

Barry Smith

Barry Smith is Senior Vice President, American Airlines Decision Technologies. He is an internationally recognized expert in the fields of yield management and reservation system design. Smith has developed many of the yield management techniques currently in use at American Airlines and pioneered the application of yield management techniques in other industries.

Yield management is a process used to increase revenues by controlling the number of sales to various customer types. Within the airline industry, yield management has been described as "selling the right seats to the right customers at the right prices" (AMR 1987 annual report). Yield management was developed in the airline industry, but it has been successfully applied to the hotel, car rental, cruise line and package tour industries. Yield management is generally applied in situations where a limited inventory of services (such as airline seats) are reserved in advance by a variety of customer types. Because the value of any reservation depends on the service requested and the customer type, the service provider can increase revenues and profitability by accepting the best number of reservations from each customer type. The concepts and application of yield management will be described in the context of the airline industry. Applications to other sectors of the travel industry will then be reviewed.

Planning Functions

Yield management is the most operational aspect of the marketing planning process. For the airlines, this process consists of three steps. First, the schedule establishes what products the airline will sell. Second, the pricing structure determines how the marketplace will be segmented (using booking restrictions) and the value of each product (the fares). Third, yield management determines how much of each product will be put on the shelf for sale (the store-front is the reservation system). While the schedule and price tend to be long-term strategic decisions, yield management is an operational process. The pricing structure for a given market is generally set for a three- to six-month season. By adjusting reservation availability for each class, yield management can control the minimum price available for any itinerary for any future flight. As a result, the pricing structure can be tailored to the specific demand for every future departure of every flight.

Futurescope

Yield management—the process of controlling the number of sales to different customer types—can be the source of maximum profitability in good times and can provide the margin of safety and survival during economic downturns. Successful organizations in the travel industry will adopt some form of the strategic perspective of yield management in the future.

The objective for yield management is to determine the number and mix of reservations for each future flight that will maximize revenue and profitability. This is done in three ways. First, yield management determines how many total reservations should be sold for a future flight. This often involves overbooking to offset the effects of cancellations and no-shows. Second, yield management determines how many reservations to sell in each of the various classes. Questions such as how many first class versus coach reservations should be offered for sale, and how many within coach, how many full fare versus discount reservations should be sold are addressed. Finally, yield management determines how many reservations to make available to the various passenger itineraries on the flight. A passenger itinerary is the origin-destination market for the passenger. A given flight may serve many different markets. For example, a flight from Austin (Texas) to Dallas/Fort Worth (DFW) serves the local Austin to DFW market. It also serves Austin to any city that can be reached from DFW via connections. For example, Austin-DFW-New Orleans, Austin-DFW-Boston, Austin-DFW-London. The customers in each of these markets have widely different values to the airline.

Decision Making

Yield management decisions are made using the following process:

1. Collect and store history. For each flight, reservation booking patterns are collected at various points prior to departure. Actual traffic and revenue for departed flights are also collected and stored. These data are used to determine reservation demand and value.

2. Review current booking patterns for future flights. The number and mix of reservations booked for all future flights are reviewed. This is used to determine actual, current reservation demand and supply.

3. Forecast future passenger behavior. Forecasts of demand, cancellations, no-shows, and standbys are produced by combining data from past flight and the current conditions on future flights.

4. Produce reservation controls. Forecasts of demand are compared to the remaining available supply of seats. From this comparison, opportunities for additional revenue can be determined. Appropriate overbooking limits, discount allocations, and itinerary controls are produced.

Each of these steps can be accomplished manually or by automation in a computer system. Due to the volume of data and the complexity of the decisions, automation is necessary for all but the most basic yield management applications. Demand forecasting and reservation control generation make use of sophisticated mathematical models to estimate future customer behavior and the appropriate response to it.

Other Applications

Each of the steps described for the airline industry has application in a number of other transportation settings. In its most general form yield management involves controlling reservation sales associated with some future service resources (for example an airline seat) at a certain control point (flight number, departure date), by product type (physically different service such as first versus coach), customer type (business—full fare versus leisure— discount) and customer itinerary (origin—destination). Yield management for other industries can be categorized using similar factors (See Table 1).

For example, in the hotel industry, reservations are controlled for all dates at each location. Reservations are allocated by room type (suite, concierge, standard), rate program (rack rate, corporate, group, qualified discount) and length of stay. Car rental reservations are controlled for all future days at a rental location by car type, rate program, and length of rental. Cruise lines control reservation availability for each future sailing by berth and cabin type. Reservations are controlled for group versus individual bookings by cabin type. Discounts are generally provided through cabin upgrades. Cruise lines often provide air transportation from "gateway cities." The customer itineraries are based on the originating gateway. Pack-

Table 1   Comparison of Yield Management Applications for Various Industries

Industry	Resource	Control Point	Product	Pricing	Itinerary
Airline	Seat	Flight # Departure Date	Compartment • First • Coach	Booking class • Full fare • Discount	Origin-Destination
Hotel	Room	Location Customer arrival date	Room type • Suite • Concierge • Standard	Rate program • Rack Rate • Corporate • Qualified discount	Length of stay
Car Rental	Vehicle	Rental location Customer arrival date	Car type	Rate program • Rack Rate • Corporate • Qualified discount	Length of rental
Cruise Line	Berth	Ship Sailing date	Cabin type	Individual Group Discounts through cabin upgrades	Originating city for package customers
Package Tour	Flight Seat and room	Departure date Resort location	Room type	Individual Group	Originating city

age tour operators control reservations for all future days within a resort. Reservations are controlled by room type and gateway city. Discounts are generally provided through pricing promotions.

Strategic Uses

Yield management can provide significant revenue benefits. For a given schedule and price structure yield management can increase revenues by 5 percent to 10 percent depending on the level of demand. The measurable benefits are greatest when demand is high relative to supply, for example, high load factors for airlines, high occupancy for hotels. In situations with strong pricing competition, yield management can be the difference between survival and failure. Without yield management, a price reduction in the market place provides two unprofitable options. First, match the price reduction and risk selling too many seats/rooms at the lower price. Second, don't match and risk market share loss. Yield management provides a third alternative. Match the lower price on a portion of the inventory. Sell the lower price inventory when excess supply is available, restrict the sales of this lower price product when demand is strong.

In any industry, yield management is an integral part of the marketing process. It is more than a computer system or even a department. It is a way of doing business. The day-to-day application of yield management often involves turning away a discount reservation request long before the resource (flight or hotel) is fully booked. This generally goes against the traditional objectives of filling seats or rooms at any price. As a result, a yield management philosophy must become an integral part of the way the organization conducts its business. This requires the support of senior management and constant education of reservations and field personnel. Once successfully integrated within an organization, yield management becomes a necessary component of the marketing process.

–41–

ELECTRIC UTILITY MARKETING

Jerry J. Neal

Jerry J. Neal is Manager of Marketing Program Management at the Public Service Company of New Mexico. He has more than 20 years of experience in the electric utility industry in the areas of customer service, marketing and sales, technical analysis of residential and commercial buildings, and electric utility system engineering analysis. Neal attended the University of New Mexico, where he earned an MA in management from the Robert O. Anderson Graduate School of Management and a BS in electrical engineering. He was a founding member of the New Mexico chapter of the American Marketing Association, and later served as the chapter's second president. During his tenure as president, the chapter was named Chapter of the Year. Neal also serves as a member of the AMA's Professional Chapters Council, and is the president and owner of a utility marketing consulting business, Prescriptive Services.

Utility Marketing? Seems like an oxymoron doesn't it? It may seem odd for most that a natural monopoly industry such as the utility business, especially the electric utility business, would engage in marketing practices and follow the marketing discipline. But the electric utility business has done so, it does so today, and those utilities in the industry that survive the decade of the 1990s will continue to do so. It may be well that we spend a few moments examining the role that marketing has historically played in the electric utility business, the role it currently plays, and the role electric utilities *must allow* it to play in the rapidly approaching future.

The Historical Role

Going back to its origin, electricity was a commodity. We can call this the era of "selling to the customer." Just about all electricity could do was provide light—made possible by our friend Thomas Edison. In the early days, the term the *light company* really meant what it said. Salespeople actually went door-to-door selling the wiring, light bulbs, and installation service. In those days, marketing was no more complicated than cold-call selling. Edison's invention, the light bulb, created a market, and the "light company" sold the bulbs and the whole infrastructure to keep them burning brightly. The industry grew rapidly as more and more uses for electricity were developed. As the use of electricity began to take on multiple forms through the introduction of a myriad of electric appliances and other industrial applications sold by other industries, consumers began to abandon the thought that electricity was a commodity. In time, they began seeing electricity as a service.

The First Wake-Up Call and the Next Era

From the early days to about the mid-1970s, marketing largely remained a selling function. Added to this was the phenomena of "economies of scale," which made it more profitable for electric utilities to build larger and larger power plants

Futurescope

It is a new time. Even "natural monopolies," such as electric utilities, must adapt to the new day of proactive marketing, of listening to and responding appropriately to the customer. Those that adjust to their new environment and develop a customer-sensitive marketing culture throughout their organizations will survive and prosper. Those that don't will fall by the wayside.

to serve the growing marketplace at continually decreasing per unit costs, thus creating the incentive to sell even more.

But the build-and-sell frenzy changed abruptly after the first oil embargo in 1973. The embargo became the first of many wake-up calls for the industry. The embargo caused the price of generating electricity to skyrocket in just a few short years. Consumers felt it in their pocketbooks for the first time ever, and boy did they respond! They used less. They used so much less that it actually blew apart the economy-of-scale phenomena. Utilities suddenly found themselves saddled with significant amounts of very large generating plants that had no buyers: huge investment—very little return.

So the industry entered a new era of marketing. Let's call this the era of "*managing* the customer*." During this period and persisting in many utilities today, this means getting the customer to "demand" electricity when it is most beneficial for the utility. This is accomplished through pricing mechanisms and other forms of incentives which also makes it beneficial for participating customers. It works relatively well while generating assets are high-priced and plentiful. But as generating supplies deplete over time, and as new forms of competition emerge in a marketplace that has heretofore never seen competition, this era of marketing will begin to play itself out.

The New Era

Enter the new era of marketing. The era of "listening to the customer." As absurd as it may seem to those in other businesses, satisfying customer wants and needs wasn't historically necessary to survive in the electric utility business. Even though electric utilities have done the best they can to satisfy customers, actual performance from their customers' perception is that electric utilities are not doing a very good job of satisfying customer needs. Customers expect more value for the price they pay for electric service. The old business paradigm, where electric utilities are under heavy regulation and where they are "managing" the customer, doesn't provide the proper framework for giving customers more value.

But things are changing. Sweeping economic reform; regulatory, legislative, and judicial initiatives; and the rapid emergence of various forms of competition are forcing electric utilities to re-examine what role marketing plays in their future. And the news is good. There is a growing recognition that the industry is moving into a new business paradigm where marketing, true marketing, customer-focused and market-driven marketing, is the industry's only salvation. Customers are no longer captive. They have choices. And they know it. And the choices are spreading. Electric utilities that quickly adjust to these changes and embrace the challenges of this business paradigm shift will survive and prosper. The laggards will slowly wither away while watching these leading-edge utilities practice marketing at its best, just as we have seen in the telecommunications industry, the airline industry, and the banking industry.

There are nine initiatives electric utilities can follow in the decade of the 1990s to aid them in becoming value-based marketing organizations that are customer-focused and market-driven.

1. Have a Mission—a Vision

The entire business needs a vision for the future that employees can rally around. The vision must be something they can live by and fight for.

2. Carefully Examine the Current Situation

Utilities must understand their markets as well as their environment. They must thoroughly examine the current situation about the economy, competition, customer research, regulation, value-price-cost relationships, information and data producing systems, and employee skills and organization culture.

3. Develop Strategies

Based upon the situation and the vision, utilities must develop overall strategies that will point the direction for work to be done in areas such as economic development, public relations, the political arena, the regulatory arena, advertising, and new business development.

4. Segment the Market

Utility markets must be segmented in order to focus strategies and resources at homogeneous groups of customers in meaningful ways.

5. "Listen to the Customer" and Identify Wants and Needs for Each Segment

Through primary and secondary research, as well as just getting out of the office and "listening" to customers on their premises, utilities must identify the core service and the value-added attributes each segment expects.

6. Organize to Remove Barriers to Delivering Excellent Service

The old vertically aligned, bureaucratic organization won't work. Functional barriers prevent cooperation in the delivery of excellent service. Utilities must reorganize into teams that are fully equipped with staff and skill sets to deliver excellent service without having to cross functional barriers.

7. Interview and Hire the Right People

If everything is in place and utilities don't properly match the skills and attitudes needed in value-based marketing against the personnel in the organization, marketing efforts are doomed to failure. The marketing area needs the most visionary and talented people in the business.

8. Reward Employees Based on Performance Objectives They Control

Utilities must make sure objectives are clear, mutually established, and tied to compensation systems that encourage extraordinary effort and results. If the compensation system works, utilities will attract talented people and retain their best people.

9. Top Management Must Be "On the Team"

Unless top management is on the team, marketing efforts for utilities will flounder. Top management must believe in the marketing vision and prove that they believe through their involvement. A lack of conviction at the top is easily sensed by employees and can be very discouraging.

If utilities follow these nine initiatives, they will find themselves ready to face the marketing challenges of the 1990s and beyond, and position themselves to begin operating in a profit center business culture with the customer as the driver of the business.

—42—
THE CHANGING
SEASONS OF
MARKETING

Judith Waldrop

Judith Waldrop has been research editor of *American Demographics* magazine since 1987. Her writing has been honored by the American Society of Business Press Editors, the American Diabetes Association, the National Religious Public Relations Council, the National Easter Seal Society and American Association of Disability Communicators, and others. She began writing on seasonal variations in consumer markets in 1988 and this was the topic of her first book, *The Seasons of Business.* Prior to coming to *American Demographics,* Ms. Waldrop worked for ten years as a city planner. She holds an MPA from Florida Atlantic University and a BGS from Auburn University at Montgomery.

Some 160 years ago, Mardi Gras was just a bunch of drunken revelers carrying rakes and rattling cow bells. By 1990, at least seven southern states held festivities. And businesses in New Orleans raked in $480 million during their five-day celebration. The seasons of business are constantly changing. Today's new celebrations include Earth Day (1970), Grandparents' Day (1978), and Martin Luther King's Birthday (1986). They express America's increasing commitment to the environment, health, family relationships, and ethnic pride.

Old holidays, like Mother's Day, are changing, too. Only about 25 percent of Hallmark's Mother's Day cards are addressed to the traditional "Mom." The rest are addressed to aunts, stepmothers, grandmothers, sisters, friends, baby-sitters, dads who fill in for moms, and anyone else who has ever been like a mother to someone. The importance of recognizing family relationships is increasing as broken and blended families become commonplace and as working mothers grow more dependent on child-care providers.

Travel is being influenced by the same factors that are reinventing America's holidays. When Ward and June Cleaver took Wally and the Beaver on vacation, the whole family went together on a month-long summer break. But coming up with a single vacation plan is harder for dual-earner couples and parents of stepchildren. Americans now take more frequent, but shorter vacations. And the fastest-growing season for pleasure travel is winter, according to the U.S. Travel Data Center. America's increasingly mobile retired population is also pushing the trend toward year-round travel.

Some new travel trends have resulted from America's increasing ethnic pride. For instance, African-American heritage sites in Alabama, Georgia, and Tennessee are attracting a growing number of tourists. Visits are particularly high during Black History Month in February. If blacks could be encouraged to take as many

Futurescope

New holidays have emerged around America's growing ethnic populations. In the Southwest, millions of Americans celebrate the Mexican victory over the French in 1862, Cinco de May (the Fifth of May). During the 1980s, the Mexican-American population grew 53 percent, to 22 million. And this segment of the population promises to continue to grow into the 21st century, surpassing blacks to become the nation's largest minority. While ethnic celebrations have always been a part of American culture, they have never been reserved for minorities. On St. Patrick's Day, everybody's Irish. If the popularity of Cinco de Mayo spreads as rapidly as America's love of tacos and burritos, someday everyone will be Mexican on May 5.

vacations as whites, the number of adult vacationers would swell by nearly 3 million people annually.

Seasonal fluctuations create marketing opportunities. Some seasons, which appear to be related to the weather and other factors, are actually market driven. One-third of all moves take place in June, July, and August—twice the share that occur during December, January, and February. Although the school calendar and weather appear to be responsible for the summer upsurge, they are not. The elderly and parent of preschoolers are just as likely to move in the summer as people with children in school. And movers follow the same seasonal pattern whether they live in the coldest or the hottest regions of the United States.

Americans move in summer because that's when the greatest selection of housing is available. Home builders and landlords put property on the market then because they know they will draw many customers. The real winner is the seller. When a relatively high percentage of householders are looking for new housing, many shoppers come through, and suppliers gain valuable information on the true market value of their property. "Dense markets have shorter marketing periods and higher sales prices." says John L. Goodman of the Federal Reserve Board. And this advantage applies to almost any seasonal product.

Timing is different for every type of product, but it is also different for every type of customer. Two weeks before Christmas, half of Americans aged 60 and older have completed their shopping, compared with only one-third of all adults, according to the Roper Organization. One in four adults under age 30 isn't finished with holiday shopping on Christmas Eve.

Older people have the time to shop early and might want to avoid the stress of last-minute shopping. They also have enough discretionary income to take advantage of bargains whenever they find them throughout the year. But young adults have less discretionary income and live in smaller dwellings without much storage space. Friendships and relationships are also less predictable. A present purchased for a boyfriend in June could be unnecessary in December.

Marketers can't limit their advertising and promotional efforts to key months. Bicyclists, for instance, are most likely to enjoy their sport from April to October, but May and June dominate new bicycle sales to adults. Critical decisions about buying, including price and brand, are frequently made during the winter. Once the customer decides to buy, he or she acts quickly, according to an NFO survey. Thirty percent of bicyclists who have a price in mind shop less than one day before making a purchase. And 80 percent of those who have a brand in mind buy that brand. Marketers who make an impression during the winter months are rewarded in the spring.

Marketers can use knowledge about their customers to locate them during the off-season. Using data from Simmons Market Research Bureau, analysts find that alpine skiers enjoy golf, tennis and other sports during the summer months. Marketers can place advertising in the sports publications that skiers read most often. And they can design special promotions for sporting events that skiers are likely to attend during the off-season. Ski resorts can extend their season by creating summer sports programs that appeal to their winter customers.

The length of some seasons, like cold and flu season, are difficult to control. Still, advertising and pre-season discounts can convince consumers to prepare for the worst by stocking up on vitamins and medicines. And marketers can strongly influence the timing of many other marketing periods. Atlantic City first established the Miss America Pageant in 1921 to stretch its summer tourist season past Labor Day. In 1976, legalized gambling turned the city into a year-round tourist destination.

Too much seasonality can limit growth. Between 1960 and 1990, annual per-capita turkey consumption in America increased from 6 pounds per person to 18. Rapid growth like this could not have taken place if consumers continued to reserve this food for holiday meals.

The increased consumption of low-fat, low-calorie turkey is linked to America's increasing concerns about health. But consumers would not have changed their habits if it weren't for changes in the product and how it was marketed. New products, like turkey sausage, ham, and hot dogs; ground turkey; and turkey parts made it possible for Americans to adapt this healthful food to their year-round diets. And marketers used advertising and recipe offers to educate consumers about how to prepare these new foods.

Marketing takes place in a constantly changing seasonal environment with its own climate and landscape. Consumers are influenced by a combination of factors: weather, geography, tradition, and trends. Each year, they pass through the same territory, but landmarks gradually change. It is not enough to know that kids need new sneakers before school starts and umbrellas sell best when it rains. The marketer must understand how the consumer's total environment shapes purchasing behavior.

Section VII

Information Collection and Analysis

Making sense of the numbers: it has always been problematic and always been key to marketing success. Yet, as the articles in this section demonstrate, increased sophistication has and will enable marketers to measure customer reaction and respond to it more quickly and effectively than ever.

The retail store level—where customer, product and marketer meet face to face and the decision to buy or not to buy is made—has always been the "trenches" of sales and marketing. In "Efficient Consumer Response: Retailers' New Competitive Weapon," Doug Adams outlines the ways that new measurement technologies will determine which marketers know their customers best and prosper in the new century. Of course, interpretation of information will be key, and in "Multivariate Statistics," Gary Mullet describes the advances, current and future, that will make analysis and interpretation more efficient, effective, and useful. Usefulness implies needs, and in "Marketing Dialects," Frank Cespedes uses the metaphor of different languages and dialects to outline the problem of the different and sometimes conflicting information needs of different marketing groups and points the way to the need for better integration as key to solving these "unspoken" problems.

—43—

EFFICIENT CONSUMER RESPONSE

Retailers' New Competitive Weapon

Doug Adams

Doug Adams is president of the Efficient Consumer Response (ECR) and Operational Applications Division of Nielsen Marketing Research NA. As such, he is responsible for developing and directing the company's ECR activities, including designing and implementing strategies and tactics, products and services, and marketing. He is also responsible for several specific product areas, including coordinating daily store-level data acquisition and processing, ECR software applications, and logistic management systems. Adams has been a regular speaker at industry conferences in the United States and Europe. He holds a bachelor's degree in economics and an M.B.A. in finance and marketing from Emory University.

After several decades of strong dominance, the supermarket industry faces significant new challenges as it faces the 21st century. Over the long run, competition is good for the industry because it forces a reevaluation of the traditional ways and generates creative thinking for the new challenges.

Alternative-format retailers are grabbing market share from supermarkets by focusing on satisfying consumer needs and driving costs from the supply side of the business equation. Critical to their competitive gains has been their willingness to embrace new technology and to form mutually beneficial strategic alliances with suppliers. Equally important has been a commitment to flow-through, a concept that calls for quickly moving the right products to the right stores in the right quantities at the right time, with minimal warehousing and inventory costs.

Accurate and timely electronic information about consumer purchases fuels this process. Checkout scanners record the UPC bar codes that identify individual products, and retailers then use third-party software applications to integrate scanning data with demographic data, pricing/promotion data, and other market research to gain insights into customers' purchasing behavior. Meanwhile, trading partners place orders, send shipping documents, and relay invoices and payments through electronic data interchange (EDI). During the last 20 years, the grocery industry has seen its productivity growth fall behind other retail trade channels' as mass-merchandise retailers have matched, and in some cases surpassed, supermarkets' technological lead in bar-coded product identification and the use of EDI.

The creation of different trade classes has led to increasingly adversarial relationships between supermarkets and their suppliers, with each side seeking to increase its profits, often at the expense of the other. Steady increases in trade promotion spending have spawned excessive inventories and product assortments based more on financial imperatives than on consumer demand.

Alarmed by the growth of the alternative-format retailers, grocery industry leaders in 1992 formed a task force to analyze the grocery supply chain and its trade practices, to study the practices of other retail trade channels, and to develop

Futurescope

Those at the forefront of the Efficient Consumer Response (ECR) movement now will be the grocery industry's leaders at the start of the 21st century, because they will know better than anyone how to satisfy customer needs while maximizing supply-chain efficiencies, minimizing inventories, and capitalizing on information, technology, and applications. The new century will require these forward-looking strategies as a condition of survival.

recommendations for making supermarkets more competitive. Known as the Efficient Consumer Response Working Group, the task force enlisted the assistance of a management consulting firm, Kurt Salmon Associates, which had been instrumental in the development and implementation of the Quick Response process used by mass merchandisers to reduce inventory costs and to speed products to retail shelves.

The result was a report unveiled in early 1993 calling for an industry-wide commitment to Efficient Consumer Response (ECR), a strategy in which distributors and suppliers work closely together to reduce costs within the supply chain and to bring better value to the grocery consumer. The report identified multiple opportunities for cost reduction through ECR. However, it said these savings could be realized only if trading partners transformed win/lose adversarial relationships into win/win strategic alliances, and only if they capitalized on scanning data analyses and EDI to maximize market intelligence and to create a timely, paperless flow of information with efficient product flow from the manufacturing line to the checkout counter.

The Principles of ECR

ECR is anchored by the following five guiding principles:

1. Trading partners must constantly focus on providing better value to the grocery consumer, including better product, better quality, better assortment, better in-stock service, and better convenience with less cost throughout the supply chain.

2. ECR must be driven by committed business leaders determined to profit from the replacement of the old paradigms with the win/win mutually profitable business of providing value to consumers.

3. Accurate and timely information must be used to support effective marketing, production, and logistics decisions. This information will flow externally between partners through EDI using uniform communications standards (UCS) and will internally affect the most productive and efficient use of information in a computer-based system.

4. To ensure the right product is available at the right time, product must flow with a maximization of value-adding processes from the end of production/packing to the consumer's basket.

5. A common and consistent performance measurement and reward system must be used that focuses on the effectiveness of the total system (i.e., better value through reduced costs, lower inventory, and better asset utilization), clearly identifies the potential rewards (i.e., increased revenue and profit), and promotes a mutually satisfactory sharing of the rewards.

Industry-wide application of these principles—which the task force has called for by the end of 1996—is expected to product substantial benefits, including $10 billion in supply-chain savings in the warehouse-supplied dry-grocery segment and more than $30 billion in supply-chain savings overall.

Product inventories, which typically rank second in value behind property among grocers' assets, are expected to shrink significantly, accounting for a large chunk of the cost savings under ECR. For example, dry-grocery inventories are projected to shrink 41 percent, from 104 days to 61 days, as products move faster from the production line to checkout counter. The task force predicts that these savings ultimately will be passed on to consumers, just as savings generated by the Quick Response program have been passed through in the general-merchandise segment, fueling its growth. ECR is expected to produce an average consumer price reduction of nearly 11 percent in dry groceries, which theoretically would close the price differential between supermarkets and mass merchandisers and wholesale clubs.

The Strategies of ECR

Whether the grocery industry can realize these benefits will depend largely on the successful implementation of the following four ECR strategies outlined by the task force:

1. **Efficient store assortments:** Optimize the productivity of inventories and store space at the consumer interface.

2. **Efficient replenishment:** Optimize time and cost in the replenishment system.

3. **Efficient promotion:** Maximize the total system efficiency of trade and consumer promotions.

4. **Efficient product introductions:** Maximize the effectiveness of activities for new-product development and introduction.

These strategies are aimed at producing cost savings and financial savings, which will in turn lead to consumer price reductions. Cost savings result from the elimination of activities or expenses and the better absorption of fixed or overhead costs. Financial savings stem from reducing inventory or other physical assets required to generate each dollar of consumer sales. Unlike cost savings, financial savings do not represent a direct cost reduction, but instead allow a grocery system to operate at a lower operating margin and still deliver the same return on investment for shareholders.

Cost and financial savings realized by eliminating inefficiencies in store assortments should enable grocers to reduce consumer prices 1.5 percent in the dry-grocery segment. As a result, grocers should realize increased inventory turns and increased sales and gross margin per retail square foot. More efficient product introductions are expected to produce a dry-grocery price reduction of 0.9 percent, with fewer unsuccessful introductions and better-value products.

But the most significant cost and financial savings—and subsequent consumer price reducations—are expected to accrue from maximizing the efficiencies of replenishment and promotions. Driving the savings in the replenishment area will be advances such as automated retail and warehouse ordering, implementation of flow-through logistics, reduced product damage, and reduced wholesale inventories. Collectively these innovations are expected to generate a 4.1 percent decrease in dry-grocery consumer prices.

To foster the growth of flow-through logistics in the grocery industry, Nielsen North America, Schaumburg, Illinois, has joined forces with a business partner to develop a plan that calls for replacing retailers' warehouses with flow-through distribution centers owned and operated by independent third parties. Similar to flow-through distribution centers now operated by some mass merchandisers, these centers would operate on a just-in-time basis with little inventory, funneling products to retailers from suppliers at a significantly lower cost than retailers would incur through their own warehouses. In the promotions area, new efficiencies in warehousing, transportation, and administration, coupled with reduced forward-buy and supplier inventories, are expected to yield a 4.3 percent reduction in prices for dry-grocery items.

Retailers and suppliers are expected to share almost equally in the cost and financial savings produced by ECR, with suppliers realizing about 54 percent of total system savings (including 7 percent from financial savings) and retailers realizing about 46 percent (including 14 percent from financial savings). The greater savings realized by suppliers reflects the fact that they incur a much greater percentage of supply-chain costs (70 percent) than does the retailer (30 percent).

In addition to the cost and financial savings and the nearly 11 percent reduction in consumer prices for dry-grocery items engendered by ECR, it is likely to produce other less tangible but still important benefits for suppliers, retailers, and consumers. Suppliers should enjoy reduced out-of-stocks, enhanced brand integrity, and improved distributor relationships. Retailers should realize increased consumer loyalty, better consumer knowledge, and improved supplier relationships. And consumers should benefit from increased choice and shopping convenience, reduced out-of-stock items, and fresher products.

Becoming Consumer-Driven

At the heart of the four strategies of ECR is the consumer. What he or she wants and buys, where they buy it, how often, and in what quantities are the key factors driving store assortments, replenishment, promotions, and new products. And consumer satisfaction must be the ultimate goal of ECR strategies in each of these areas. Quite simply, the suppliers and retailers that understand consumer needs most thoroughly will stand the best chance of implementing ECR successfully.

As the grocery industry commits itself to ECR, growing numbers of retailers and suppliers are striving to become more customer-driven by simultaneously adopting an innovative marketing strategy known as *category management*. Rooted in the belief that today's new-product explosion has made strategic management by item too impractical and strategic management by department too unfocused, category management is a process that involves managing product categories as business units and customizing each category's product mix, merchandising, and promotions to satisfy customer needs on a store-by-store basis.

The lifeblood of category management is market intelligence. It stems from technological advances, including electronic checkout scanners, decision support systems, powerful computer applications, and demographic databases. Software applications then produce information for analyzing pricing, promotions, and shelf space. The information yields marketing knowledge, which, in turn, leads to strategies, tactics, and action. Category management can be used as a tool throughout the ECR process, beginning with maximizing the efficiency of product assortments at individual stores by tailoring them to customer demand, and continuing through the development of efficient promotion, replenishment, and new-product strategies.

Third-party software applications that figure prominently in category management—including promotion-planning programs, advanced forecasting systems, and modeling and decision-support systems—enable retailers and suppliers to factor current price changes, shelf-space allocations, promotion data, household-panel data, and other data into ECR decisions, instead of relying solely on historical order-system data when making pivotal decisions about replenishment and inventories.

This allows retailers and suppliers to optimize their merchandising/marketing mix of individual items and individual stores. It also enables them to focus more on consumer demand when making such decisions, a consideration that often finishes behind financial imperatives as retailers strive to capitalize on forward buys and diverting practices that historically have caused production inefficiencies for suppliers and excess inventories for retailers. But more importantly, the information, technology, and applications that drive category management provide a solid grasp of the demand side of the grocery business equation. By providing knowledge about normal shelf turns and promotion effects, category management also provides a dynamic link to the supply side of the equation, creating an opportunity to improve the efficiency of how products are moved to the consumer.

How to Get ECR Started

ECR cannot be implemented in one fell swoop. For most companies with up-to-date information systems, it requires a continuous incremental investment over 2–4 years. A moderate investment of seed money the first year should be enough to create a self-funding program through cost savings and inventory reductions. Sometimes significant savings can be realized without any major capital investments. For example, joint supplier/retailer teams working on truck-loading, handling, and deduction improvement projects have produced cost savings as high as 0.3 percent of sales at some companies.

People costs often are the biggest ECR expense. The process requires ongoing education and training at all levels to help employees adapt to new roles and to let go of familiar habits. It also requires the implementation of new performance measures for business units and individuals.

The best way to implement ECR at your company is to launch three concurrent programs: create a climate for change, select partners for ECR alliances, and develop an information technology investment program.

Create a Climate for Change

This involves changing the perception of suppliers or customers as adversaries. You should anticipate that this will take longer than will any other part of ECR. It will require the demonstrated commitment of your company's leaders, coupled with effective communication and education programs and new performance measurement and reward systems.

Select Partners for ECR Alliances

Start with 2–4 alliances. Set up a one-day meeting to discuss ECR and to develop a game plan. Establish a few joint task forces to work on projects known to generate significant paybacks, such as eliminating invoice deductions, improving truck loading and unloading efficiency, and reducing product damage. Success in these areas will provide a foundation of trust and confidence for future cooperative efforts.

Develop an Information Technology Investment Program

Although ECR can be implemented without a huge, one-time investment, the companies with the strongest information technology will be the big winners under ECR. Those now at the forefront of the ECR movement envision an almost paperless, fully integrated business information system linking them with their business partners within five years.

No company can realize the full benefits of ECR unless a majority of its suppliers or customers are involved in the process. For example, a retailer that has invested in EDI will realize little return until its suppliers do the same. Critical mass is achieved when one-quarter to one-third of a company's trading partners have adopted a specific element of ECR, and major benefits begin to accrue when one-half to one-third of a company's trading partners have come online with the process.

With ECR gaining momentum across the grocery industry, it's clear that companies that adopt ECR early will gain a significant competitive advantage over others. If the experience of mass merchandisers with Quick Response is a barometer, ECR will cause rapid changes once it takes root in the grocery industry.

—44—
MULTIVARIATE STATISTICS

Gary M. Mullet

Gary M. Mullet, Ph.D., is President and Principal of Gary Mullet Associates, Inc., a consulting and statistical data processing firm concentrating on marketing research. His work experience includes time with Sophisticated Data Research and Burke Marketing Research. He has taught at the Universities of Cincinnati and Michigan, and at Georgia Institute of Technology. He has published several articles on statistics and marketing research and is active in various professional organizations as a reviewer and a presenter. His degrees are from Central Michigan University, North Carolina State University, and the University of Michigan. His clients include both marketing research suppliers and end-users of research.

Although not a formal, official definition, in the discussion that follows, multivariate statistics will be looked at as analytical methods that are widely used in marketing research, but that cannot be performed with a standard, off-the-shelf crosstabulation package. Thus, for example, we will not talk about independent groups (or cells) t-tests for differences in means, because most crosstab packages can do this type of analysis. Also, be aware that some crosstab packages will be able to help the user perform some of the techniques covered here.

Common Multivariate Tools

With any and all of the techniques discussed here, the user will have to make decisions about significance levels, decisions about which of several methods to use within the technique, decisions about handling item nonresponse, and several others. These will be ignored, because the intent is to give the reader the flavor of each of several multivariate tools without bogging anyone down in excessive statistical jargon.

Factor Analysis

One widely used technique is factor analysis. Factor analysis puts questions together into sets called *factors*. The grouping is usually done by analyzing the correlation patterns between all answers across all of the respondents in a study. Thus, you might see all of the statements having to do with convenience, and no others, together in a single factor. Likewise, all of the statements having to do with price/value would probably be in a single factor. It is not uncommon to end up with only one-third as many factors, or fewer, as the number of original questions. Then subsequent interpretation of the results of a study can be much easier, because the analyst is dealing with a smaller number of variables. The trade-off, however,

---

Futurescope

The growth in the use of multivariate statistics by the marketing-research industry has accelerated greatly during the past few years. This growth is due to decreasing prices for increasing computing power, wider availability of computer software, and a higher knowledge and awareness level of these particular statistical tools among marketing researchers. The latter comes both from graduate schools and colleges, as well as seminars and tutorials. The competitive marketplace of the 21st century will require as much analytic firepower as the marketer can bring to bear.

is in the loss of variance explained by using factors as opposed to using the original rating data.

Factor analytic results are frequently used as inputs into regression analysis or cluster analysis. They are also used to help interpret the "true" dimensions (constructs) of the product or service being rated. Frequently, factor results are used to reduce the number of scales/ratings in future studies, assuming that the items in a given factor would continue to be correlated in the future. Among other types of studies, factor analysis is sometimes used on customer satisfaction studies when customers evaluate a large number of attributes.

Cluster Analysis

Cluster analysis is similar in concept to factor analysis, except in cluster analysis it is respondents who are being put into homogeneous groups or segments by the similarity of their answers to the basis questions. Inputs into cluster analysis can be respondent scores from factor analysis or the original ratings data itself. Some cluster programs will assign respondents to segments on the basis of their answers to a series of categorical questions or even yes-no items from a checklist, such as a listing of adjectives that respondents think do or do not apply to a product concept.

In any case, the objective of the analysis is to put a given respondent into a cluster comprised of other, similar respondents. Those who give substantively different answers will be placed into different clusters. The toughest decision for the analyst is generally to determine how many clusters are appropriate. Frequently, two or more possible solutions (e.g., both 4 segments and 5 segments) are used as banner points for further data tabulation to help make a final decision. The results of cluster analysis are often used for segmentation marketing, in its broadest sense. They also may serve as inputs into perceptual mapping.

Regression Analysis

Regression analysis has probably been used the longest in marketing research. Where factor analysis and cluster analysis operate on all of the designated variables (ratings, attitudes, behaviors, etc.) simultaneously, regression analysis requires one, and only one, of the variables to be designated as the dependent or criterion variable. Frequently, this will be overall opinion of a product or concept, purchase intent, actual purchase, or some other such variable. Regression analysis will build an equation that relates to other variables chosen, called *independent* or *predictor variables,* to that criterion variable. The equation, at the discretion of the analyst, can include all of the possible independent variables or only a statistically significant subset. It is also possible, if desired, to look at the relationship of the criterion to a designated set of independent variables, irrespective of statistical significance. This makes sense if in the latter set are all controllable variables in a marketing strategy. There are a variety of statistics that will help the user to determine which equation relating the dependent and independent variables is, in some sense, the "best" one.

The independent variables in regression are frequently ratings themselves, or they can be factor scores from a factor analysis. Factor scores will be fewer than the original number of ratings scales and are orthogonal (this helps in the computations and interpretation, to a degree). Regression is widely used in customer satisfaction measurement. It is also used to determine which product attributes are "drivers" of overall product opinion in concept tests, taste tests, in-home product use tests, and the like. Variations of regression analysis include distributed lag forecasting models and response surface analysis. The latter is a method of optimizing physical product characteristics (e.g., sugar content, weight, size, and other factors that are controllable) that will maximize respondent-stated purchase intent or some other overall measure.

Discriminant Analysis

There's not a lot of difference between regression analysis and discriminant analysis, except that in regression analysis the dependent variable is metric (overall rating, ounces consumed per week, hours spent watching TV per day, etc.), and in discriminant analysis the dependent variable is of the mutually exclusive, categorical type (e.g., brand used most often; buyer segment, possibly from cluster analysis; concept like best; etc.). Discriminant analysis will also develop a predictive relationship between the dependent variables and one or more predictors, with the same type of flexibility as a regression analysis.

The results will allow classification of respondents not included in the discriminant analysis into one of the dependent categories with an associated category. In addition to being used by the Internal Revenue Service, marketing researchers use discriminant analysis to examine for (actionable) differences between brand loyalists within a product category, to develop demographic profiles of customers versus non-customers, to do credit scoring, and to look at significantly different ratings between several concepts, among other things. Discriminant analysis results are also sometimes used in perceptual mapping.

Conjoint Analysis

Marketing researchers have been using conjoint analysis since the late 1970s. There are several conjoint analysis software algorithms available, and they seem to give highly correlated results. Thus, the conclusion will be much the same regardless of how the analysis was actually done. The input to a conjoint analysis is usually respondent-level ranking or ratings data. These are collected by showing those in the study several possible product configurations, where each consists of a combination of attributes (e.g., size, color, price), each at one of several levels (e.g., small or medium or large; red or blue or green or yellow; $1 or $1.50 or $2 or $2.50 or $3).

The particular configurations or scenarios are not chosen at random; instead, they are constructed using the principles of experimental design. The output of a conjoint analysis consists of a number, generally called a *utility,* for each level of each product attribute. The utilities are generated for each respondent and sometimes serve as the basis for cluster analysis. Utilities and their differences or ranges are important in the interpretation of conjoint studies. Recent marketing research journals seem sated with conjoint analysis articles, so only a few products in those studies will be listed: airlines' service parameters, clock radios, apartments, condominiums, STOL aircraft, automobiles, computers, package goods, and college courses. A recent variation of conjoint analysis is discrete choice modelling. As with any relatively new research offering, it has its champions and its critics.

Multidimensional Scaling/Perceptual Mapping

Multidimensional scaling and perceptual mapping are popular marketing research presentation tools. For simplicity, consider the perceptual map to be the physical result of multidimensional scaling. A perceptual map is a two-dimensional representation of a data set (on occasion, you will see a three-dimensional map, either printed or actually built by a model shop). Some maps will have arrows or vectors representing brand/product attributes and points showing the locations of the brands themselves. Some point-vector maps can be drawn by merely using crosstab tables as the inputs into the scaling algorithm, without going into the respondent-level data set. Some, of course, do use actual respondent data, rather than the summary data.

The brand locations and attribute locations are individually and jointly interpretable, irrespective of which type of point-vector map is used. So too for maps, generally from correspondence analysis, in which there are no vectors, only points. Cluster groups are frequently shown on perceptual maps to help with their interpretation and naming. As noted, discriminant-based maps are widely used. Perceptual maps, particularly color versions, make a big impact on marketing research presentations. Perceptual maps are often used in brand-positioning studies in which a large number of product ratings are collected for a number of brands within a given category.

Emerging Multivariate Tools

The multivariate methods mentioned here are probably the most widely used techniques by today's marketing research community. Certainly, other tools are gaining popularity and usefulness as statistical theory and software become more widely available. Among these techniques are confirmatory factor analysis, log-linear modelling, path analysis, structural equation modelling, and latent structure analysis, to mention just a few. The methods fleshed out here will probably not be used any less in an absolute sense for the next several years. As multivariate statistical analysis continues to grow, their relative share will probably be somewhat lessened by the continuing growth of the newer methodologies.

Finally, it should be noted that there are several software packages that will do most of the analyses discussed above. Irrespective of your hardware, you should be able to find one or more affordable packages to help. Be careful, however. Although the programs make it easy to manipulate the answers of hundreds of respondents to hundreds of questions, it is also easy to fall into the trap of doing these types of analyses just because they can be done or, even worse, doing an incorrect analysis on a given data set. There are also a variety of options within each type of analysis that should be considered carefully. Cogent interpretation of the results is also an art in itself.

—45—

MARKETING DIALECTS

Frank V. Cespedes

Frank V. Cespedes received his B.A. from the City College of New York, his M.S. from the Massachusetts Institute of Technology, and his Ph.D. from Cornell University. For fifteen years, he has been a faculty member at Harvard Business School, where he has taught in various M.B.A. and Executive Education programs. He is also a faculty partner at The Center for Executive Development in Cambridge, Massachusetts. He is the author of *Concurrent Marketing: Managing Product, Sales, and Service Linkages; Organizing and Implementing the Marketing Effort; Going to Market: Distribution Systems for Industrial Products;* as well as articles in *Harvard Business Review, California Management Review, Industrial Marketing, Marketing Research, Organization Science, Journal of Consumer Marketing, Journal of Marketing Channels, Sloan Management Review,* and other journals.

Marketing efforts typically encompass three groups: those who manage the firm's product offerings (e.g., brand or product managers); those who manage the sales channels (direct and/or indirect distribution channels); and those responsible for customer service (pre- and post-sale services of various kinds). Market factors have made better and faster coordination of these groups a prerequisite for effective marketing in many industries.

Yet these groups usually differ in terms of their roles, responsibilities, time horizons, performance criteria, and informational requirements. In marketing organizations, these differences result in a series of marketing dialects—i.e., differences in how each group hears, interprets, and articulates the voice of the customer. In turn, these marketing dialects affect the relationship between providers and users of market research.

In this brief review, three aspects of information flows within each group are discussed: (1) information priorities and, hence, the type of data tracked by each marketing unit; (2) the role of the data that is tracked; and (3) hardware and software systems used to disseminate information within and between these groups. Table 1 summarizes typical differences.

Information Priorities

Product management views data about assigned products and pertinent markets (usually defined in terms of consumer segments or, in industrial firms, applications across geographical boundaries) as its highest information priorities. Sales management views timely information about geographically defined markets, specific accounts within those markets, and the activities of resellers as priority data. Service managers seek information about both products and accounts, but in terms that typically differ from the categorizations most salient to product and sales units. An executive at a research firm describes common differences in this way:

Futurescope

When it comes to information needs, the different functional areas in marketing operations seem to speak different languages. As the 21st century opens an era of increasing internationalization, the notion of different languages achieves additional force. Information systems in coming years must strive for an integrated, cross-functional infrastructure to promote a common language for efficient problem solving across the organization and around the globe.

Table 1   Typical Differences between Marketing Groups

Product Management	Field Sales	Customer Service
Roles and responsibilities:		
Operate across geographical territories with specific product responsibilities	Operate within geographical territories, with specific account assignments	Operate within geographical territories with multiple product/ account assignments
Time horizons driven by:		
• Product development and introduction cycles • Internal planning and budgeting processes	• Selling cycles at multiple accounts • External buying processes	• Product installation/ maintenance cycles • Field service processes
Key performance criteria:		
Performance measures based on profit-and-loss and market-share metrics	Measures based primarily on annual, quarterly, or monthly sales volume	Measures vary, but typically "customer satisfaction" and cost efficiencies
Information flows:		
Data priorities: Aggregate data about products and markets (defined in terms of user segments)	**Data priorities:** Disaggregated data about geographical markets, specific accounts, and resellers	**Data priorities:** Disaggregated data about product usage at accounts
Key data uses: Role of data makes compatibility with internal planning and budgeting categories a criterion of useful information	**Key data uses:** Role of data makes compatibility with external buyers' categories important: "timely" data as a function of varied selling cycles at assigned accounts	**Key data uses:** Role of data makes compatibility with relevant technical vocabularies a criterion of useful information
Information systems: Often incompatible with sales and service systems	**Information systems:** Often incompatible with product and service systems	**Information systems:** Often incompatible with product and sales systems

Source: Frank V. Cespedes, "Market Research and Marketing Dialects," *Marketing Research* 5 (Spring 1993), 290.

Product managers tend to synthesize the information they receive; they're looking for commonalities across the data because they naturally think in terms of segments—or what seems common to aggregate groups of customers. Sales managers tend to disaggregate the information they receive, and look for exceptions—why account X differs from account Y—because they sell to specific customers, not "segments." Service most often feels a *lack* of pertinent information, and wants data about products or sales in terms of its delivery, installation, or maintenance implications—information rarely contained in the product literature, call reports, or other data that service typically receives.

In most companies, accounting systems track costs primarily by product categories (rather than, say, customer or channel categories). Also, market research typically reports through the product-marketing organization and research funds come from the marketing budget. Hence, it is product managers' priorities that drive the kinds of data and research reports routinely available to sales and service units. However, the result is often a gap between the aggregate data most meaningful to product-planning activities and the disaggregated data most meaningful to account- or region-specific selling and service activities.

Among other things, these differing information priorities mean that product, sales, and service managers often meet to discuss customer-related issues on a reactive, rather than proactive, basis. Further, each group often arrives at such meetings with ideas based on different data sources and with different assumptions about who "the customer" is. In practice, it is difficult to integrate entrenched ideas under such circumstances.

Information Uses

The role of information also differs among these marketing units.

Product managers typically need data relevant to product development, costing, and pricing decisions. More than sales or service managers, product managers work through the medium of formal presentations as part of their firms' planning processes. Hence, compatibility with the *selling* firm's budgeting vocabulary is often an important criterion of useful data.

Sales managers need data relevant to different customers. Hence, compatibility with multiple *buying* vocabularies and data categories is important to sales managers. In addition, the varied, less formal, and often time-constrained contexts of sales calls make "a few key points" a criterion of useful information for sales personnel.

Service personnel often deal with customer personnel on a wider basis than their product or sales colleagues. Especially in industrial firms, field maintenance and installation responsibilities make detailed data about product specifications and data requirements important. But, in contrast to the data priorities of product or sales units, compatibility with relevant technical and/or logistical vocabularies at customers are key criteria of useful service information.

These differences can create transmission problems in dissemination of market information. A sales manager notes:

> The biggest frustration is lack of timely information. And "timely" means data relevant to current selling efforts. The information is not useful if it arrives too late to be used in our customers' budgeting cycles.

A product manager in the same firm provides a complementary perspective:

> We spend considerable effort gathering and writing-up product and competitive information, send out that information, and reps call a week later for the same information. This takes time away from other important things.

Such comments reflect different information usage cycles. Product managers must gather and present data to and from a variety of functional areas. Such data are often assembled for use in the company's budgeting process, which, in many multiproduct firms, must adhere to a fairly rigid schedule. At packaged-goods firms, for example, the annual marketing planning process takes months, during which time brand managers are often fully occupied and so less responsive to field requests for information. By contrast, the timing of sales' and service's information needs is irregular, less capable of being scheduled, and generated (in sales' eyes at least) by an "urgent" customer need. For marketing researchers, these varying information usage situations become more important as short-cycle times and first-mover advantages become growing aspects of competitive strategy.

Information Systems

In marketing, the value of information is ultimately tied to its use in influencing buyer-seller exchange. But in many firms, information systems in product, sales, and service units have, over time, become fragmented and often technically incompatible with each other. In turn, separate systems and databases result in different (and often conflicting) assumptions and categories about customers. Meanwhile, competitive developments require faster assimilation and integration of data captured via these systems.

In some consumer-goods firms, for example, trade spending is captured via three incompatible information systems lodged in brand, sales, and logistics units and can only be aggregated at the national level across product groups. For these firms, specifying promotional paybacks in terms of class-of-trade or account is often impossible or requires time frames far in excess of the relevant selling cycles. Yet, as one executive notes,

> This data are crucial if Sales is to generate profitable volume. As the trade changes, the field will have more control over local promotion expenditures and must understand the ROI implications.

In addition, these technology issues often inadvertently exacerbate conflicts among these marketing units. As one manager comments:

> When disagreements are argued via print-outs from different spreadsheets, people start referring to "the facts" and the tone easily becomes sarcastic and accusatory on each side.

These marketing dialects illustrate an important dimension of coordination and an increasingly important role for marketing researchers working in conjunction with IS departments. Without a common information infrastructure, a frequent prescription for cross-functional collaboration—"more communication" via multifunctional teams or more task force meetings—can mean more finger pointing, not joint problem solving. Conversely, as firms face greater customization requirements across more segments, creating a common language among these groups becomes a key challenge for the organization in general and a key task for marketing researchers in particular.

For Further Reading

Albaum, Gerald, "Horizontal Information Flow: An Exploratory Study," *Journal of the Academy of Management* 7 (Winter 1964), 21–23.

Barabba, Vincent P., and Gerald Zaltman, *Hearing the Voice of the Market* (Boston, Mass.: Harvard Business School Press, 1991).

Cespedes, Frank V., "Market Research and Marketing Dialects," *Marketing Research* 5 (Spring 1993), 26–34.

Hodock, Calvin L., "The Decline and Fall of Marketing Research in Corporate America," *Marketing Research* 3 (June 1991), 12–22.

Kaplan, Robert S. "The Evolution of Management Accounting," *Accounting Review* 17 (July 1984), 404–407.

Kinnear, Thomas C., and Ann R. Root, *Survey of Marketing Research* (Chicago: American Marketing Association, 1988).

McKinnon, Sharon M., and William J. Bruns, Jr.., *The Information Mosaic* (Boston, Mass.: Harvard Business School Press, 1992).

Section VIII
Total Quality Management and the Future of Marketing

Quality has probably been the most potent concern in all of management in recent years for one simple reason: Customers have demanded it. And marketing departments have been in the forefront of responding to the challenge. In "Quality Management in Marketing," Philip Crosby outlines the basic challenges in implementing quality-conscious marketing programs and the risks of not doing so. John Hauser extends the discussion of Crosby's article in "Quality Function Deployment," analyzing the many factors that will lead to success in all operations of an organization. In "ISO 9000," Harold Steudel and Michael Scherman outline the factors that will enable an organization to meet international quality standards in their operations. How does one reach top-quality standards in one's marketing? Allan Magrath describes the process of mapping one's processes and operations in "Zero-Defect Marketing." And in "Benchmarking," C. Jackson Grayson outlines a key planning tool for achieving total-quality functions throughout a marketing organization.

–46–

QUALITY MANAGEMENT IN MARKETING

Philip B. Crosby

Philip B. Crosby worked for 27 years as a quality management professional for Martin Marietta and ITT. He is the author of *Cutting the Cost of Quality, Quality Is Free,* and *Completeness: Quality for the 21st Century.* He is featured in a weekly commentary, "On Improvement," on USA News' "First Business" television program.

Quality management is all about routinely delivering to customers the exact product or service they have been promised and doing everything right the first time in the process. The goals of quality management are to help a company cause its employees to be successful, cause its suppliers to be successful, and cause its customers to be successful. I call that completeness. Marketing is all about figuring out who can be a customer, determining exactly what they want, and making it possible for them to acquire that product or service with no hassle, and then doing it again.

Marketing and quality are a powerhouse combination for anyone willing to understand what quality really is and how to cause it to come about. First of all, we must have a definition of quality that we can communicate and measure. Results come from our relationship with customers, employees, and suppliers. We must be able to tell them what has to occur, and we must be able to measure the results in order to get better all the time.

When marketing determines the customer's requirements for a product or service, that description must be communicated to everyone. They in turn translate those specifics into requirements that provide direction for their area of operation. Because the entire company's activities are shaped by what comes from marketing, we must be certain that we take the stating of requirements seriously. If everyone conforms to those requirements, then the product or service will be exactly what it is supposed to be. Thus the definition of quality becomes "conformance to requirements." Everyone involved acts to produce what marketing has found to be a customer's desire. As that desire changes over time, the requirements are improved in order to meet the new needs.

The thrust of all management action in a quality-oriented community is toward prevention rather than correction. Learning to conform to requirements is called zero defects. The measurement of quality then becomes the price of nonconformance (PONC). Because management relates primarily to financial measurements, this places quality in a primary position of commitment. Companies that do not take quality seriously spend 25 percent of their revenues and more doing things wrong, over and over. All that money is available for other uses if we can learn to manage quality properly.

Futurescope

As we look at the world of business today, we see national borders blurring; suppliers and customers are everywhere. Lurking right beside them are our competitors. In business the race is not always to the swift, but that is the way to bet. The company that knows where customers are going and can supply them with the ever-changing needs of the trip in the 21st century will be the victor.

Figure 1   The Eternally Successful Organization™ Grid

	COMATOSE	INTENSIVE CARE	PROGRESSIVE CARE	HEALING	WELLNESS
QUALITY	Nobody does anything right around here. *Price of Nonconformance = 33%*	We finally have a list of customer complaints. *Price of Nonconformance = 28%*	We are beginning a formal Quality Improvement Process. *Price of Nonconformance = 20%*	Customer complaints are practically gone. *Price of Nonconformance = 13%*	People do things right the first time routinely. *Price of Nonconformance = 3%*
GROWTH	Nothing ever changes. *Return after tax = nil*	We bought a turkey. *Return after tax = nil*	The new product isn't too bad. *Return after tax = 3%*	The new group is growing well. *Return after tax = 7%*	Growth is profitable and steady. *Return after tax = 12%*
CUSTOMERS	Nobody ever orders twice. *Customer complaints on orders = 63%*	Customers don't know what they want. *Customer complaints on orders = 54%*	We are working with customers. *Customer complaints on orders = 26%*	We are making many defect-free deliveries. *Customer complaints on orders = 9%*	Customer needs are anticipated. *Customer complaints on orders = 0%*
CHANGE	Nothing ever changes. *Changes controlled by Systems Integrity = 0%*	Nobody tells anyone anything. *Changes controlled by Systems Integrity = 2%*	We need to know what is happening. *Changes controlled by Systems Integrity = 55%*	There is no reason for anyone to be surprised. *Changes controlled by Systems Integrity = 85%*	Change is planned and managed. *Changes controlled by Systems Integrity = 100%*
EMPLOYEES	This place is a little better than not working. *Employee turnover = 65%*	Human Resources has been told to help employees. *Employee turnover = 45%*	Error Cause Removal programs have been started. *Employee turnover = 40%*	Career path evaluations are implemented now. *Employee turnover = 7%*	People are proud to work here. *Employee turnover = 2%*

Source: Reprinted from *The Eternally Successful Organization*, ©1988 Philip B. Crosby. Reprinted with permission.

The analogy for understanding quality in a company is wellness. Personal wellness is aimed at preventing illness or disability in the individual. We have learned that taking care of ourselves, exercising, not smoking, handling stress, and eating right extends life. The same is true with organizations. The Eternally Successful Organization Grid (Figure 1).will help readers examine their own company's status. The grid is just to help you understand the idea of wellness and how it applies in work life.

If the marketing function wants the company to stay well and grow, it must recognize its unique position in that regard. My experience has been that marketing people often consider themselves not to be an integral part of the producing part of the organization. One class I had, consisting of 22 marketing directors, asked me why I was talking with the victims, rather than the muggers. As we started to discuss their opportunity to have an effect on internal operations, they became much more interested.

Change cannot happen unless every person involved wants it to happen. The ball must be passed quickly and surely. The "wellness" part of the ESO grid lays that out. Creating that kind of work environment is a purposeful task, and marketing needs to be the catalytic agent. They need to get in there and help quality become the fabric of the organization.

To accomplish this, the marketing operation must examine itself and make certain that it has incorporated the concepts of quality management into its way of life. Are things routinely done right the first time? Is growth always profitable? Are the customer's needs anticipated? Is change managed and caused? Are employees proud to work there? It does no good to complain about the inadequacies of the rest of the organization. What they need in order to change is a good example, a role model. What better place to begin than marketing?

—47—

QUALITY FUNCTION DEPLOYMENT

John R. Hauser

John R. Hauser is the Kirin Professor of Marketing at Massachusetts Institute of Technology's Sloan School of Management. He is the head of Sloan's Marketing Group, co-director of Sloan's International Center for Research on the Management of Technology, and Editor-in-Chief of *Marketing Science*. Dr. Hauser is the co-author of two textbooks, *Design and Marketing of New Products* and *Essentials of New Product Managment*, and two computer-based texts/software packages, *Applying Marketing Management* and *Enterprise: An Integrated Management Exercise*, and has published more than 40 scientific articles. In addition to writing, teaching, and researching, Dr. Hauser has also served as a consultant to leading corporations in many industries.

Quality Function Deployment (QFD) was developed in 1972 at Mitsubishi's Kobe shipyard, brought to the United States by Ford and Xerox in 1986, and has been adopted widely by Japanese, U.S., and European firms. In some applications, it has reduced design time by 40 percent and design costs by 60 percent, while maintaining and enhancing design quality. QFD helps an interfunctional team of marketing, R&D, manufacturing, and sales work together to focus on product development. It provides procedures and processes to enhance communication by focusing on the language of the customer.

QFD uses four "houses" to integrate the informational needs of the product development team. Applications begin with the first house, the House of Quality (HOQ), which is shown conceptually in Figure 1. Together the team uses the HOQ to understand the voice of the customer and to translate it to the voice of the engineer.

The Voice of the Customer

Identifying Customer Needs

A customer need is a description, in the customer's own words, of the benefit that he, she, or they want fulfilled by the product or service. For example, spirometry (a medical instrument for measuring lung capacity) users state needs such as that the product is "affordable," "easy to hold," "easy to clean," and provides "convenient-sized output."

Normally, discussions with customers identify 100–400 customer needs including basic needs (what the customer just assumes a spirometer will do), articulated needs (what the customer will tell you that he, she, or they want the spirometer

---

Futurescope

The most definitive study to date on Quality Function Deployment (QFD) in America (Griffin, 1992) suggests that the greatest impact of QFD has been the enhancement of the product development process so that it is more effective in the long term. Product development for the 21st century will be most effective when the marketing, R&D, manufacturing, and engineering functions cooperate and when they understand one another. QFD enhances communication by providing the vehicle for communication. QFD enhances market success by ensuring that each of these functions is focused on providing benefits to the customer.

Figure 1 The House of Quality

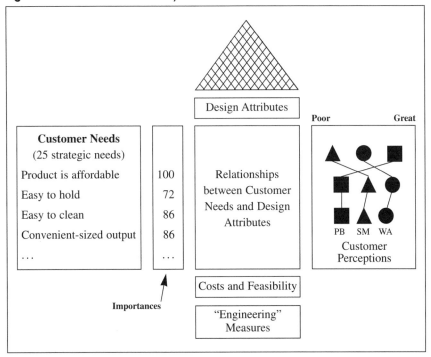

Reprinted with permission, *Sloan Management Review.*

to do), and excitement needs (those needs, which, if they were fulfilled, would delight and surprise the customer). However it is difficult for a team to work with 100–400 customer needs simultaneously.

Structuring the Needs

To make customer needs manageable, they are structured into a hierarchy. The primary need, also known as strategic needs, are generally the 5–10 top-level needs that set the strategic direction for the product. For example, "easy to use" is a strategic needs for spirometry. Secondary needs, also known as tactical needs, are elaborations of the primary needs—each primary need is usually elaborated into 3–10 secondary needs. These needs indicate more specifically what can be done to fulfill the corresponding strategic (primary) need. For example, "easy to use" is elaborated to "easy to set up the first time," "easy to operate," "fast to use," and "easy to calibrate." In most cases the secondary needs are themselves elaborated to very detailed tertiary needs. Such tertiary needs indicate specifically how the design team can fulfill the secondary needs.

Importances of the Needs

Customers want their needs fulfilled, but some needs have higher priorities than others. These priorities help the QFD team make decisions that balance the cost of fulfilling a need and the benefit to the customer. For example, if it is equally costly to fulfill two needs, then the need that the customer rates as more important should be given higher priority. For example, when designing a spirometer, Puritan-Bennett measured importances on a 100-point scale.

Customer Perceptions

Customer perceptions describe how customers evaluate competitive products in terms of the product or service's abilities to fulfill the customer needs. By understanding which products fulfill customer needs best, how well those customer needs are fulfilled, and whether there are any gaps between the best product and the firm's current product, the QFD team provides goals and identifies opportunities for product design.

The Voice of the Engineer

Design Attributes

To fulfill customer needs, the product (or service) must fulfill measurable requirements. For example, if a spirometry system provides hard-copy output, then design attributes might include resolution, fade resistance, paper loading time, printing noise, and paper-feed failure rates. These design measures are listed at the top of the house. They are measured in physical measurement units that become targets for an R&D design. However, they are not product solutions. Solutions come in the second house of QFD. If solutions are specified too early, the R&D process becomes constrained to existing solutions. New, creative directions might be missed.

Engineering Measures

Just as the design team measures competitive products with respect to customer needs, so does the team measure competitive products on the physical units specified by the design attributes.

Relationship Matrix

The QFD team judges which design attributes influence which customer needs. Each element of the relationship matrix indicates how much (if at all) each design attribute affects each customer need. The idea is to specify the strongest relationships, leaving most of the matrix (60–70 percent) blank.

Roof Matrix

Finally, the roof matrix, shown as cross-hatched lines in Figure 1, quantifies the physical interrelations among the design attributes.

Other Estimates

The team often estimates costs, feasibility, and technical difficulty for changes in each of the design attributes.

References

Griffin, Abbie, "Evaluating QFD's Use in U.S. Firms as a Process for Developing Products," *Journal of Product Innovation Management* (September 1992), 171–187.

——————and John R. Hauser, "The Voice of the Customer," *Marketing Science* (Winter 1993), 1–27.

Hauser, John R., "How Puritan-Bennett Used the House of Quality," *Sloan Management Review* 34, no. 3 (Spring 1993), 61–70.

—————— and Don P. Clausing, "The House of Quality," *Harvard Business Review* (May-June 1988), 63–73.

King, Robert, *Better Designs in Half the Time: Implementing Quality Function Deployment (QFD) in America* (Lawrence, Mass.: G.O.A.L., Inc, 1987).

Sullivan, Lawrence P., "Quality Function Deployment," *Quality Progress* 19, no. 6 (June 1986), 39–50.

–48–
ISO 9000

Harold J. Steudel and Michael V. Scherman

Harold J. Steudel, Ph.D., P.E., is president and founder of H.J. Steudel & Associates, Inc., an international consulting company. In addition, he is a professor of industrial engineering at the University of Wisconsin–Madison, where he is active in research and teaching and serves as the convener for the Quality Engineering Program. He has more than 40 published papers and is author of *Manufacturing in the Nineties: How to Become a Mean, Lean, World-Class Competitor.*

Michael V. Scherman is an engineering consultant at H.J. Steudel & Associates, Inc., where he is involved in training and implementing systems for quality and productivity improvement. He earned a B.S. degree in industrial engineering and an M.S. degree in manufacturing systems engineering from the University of Wisconsin–Madison.

The role of quality as a competitive issue in the global marketplace is clearly evident by what many international quality standards leaders refer to as the "ISO 9000 phenomenon." The impact of adoption of the ISO 9000 series as the accepted standard of quality system requirements for both quality product assessment and third-party registration is unprecedented in modern history. In only six years from the initial publication in 1987, more than 60 countries have adopted the five standards in the series—ISO 9000, ISO 9001, ISO 9002, ISO 9003, and ISO 9004—as their national standards. In the same period, more than 40,000 companies' quality-assurance systems have received third-party registration to ISO 9001, ISO 9002, or ISO 9003.[1] Because few U.S. companies became "ISO 9000 conscious" before 1990–1991, less than 250 U.S. sites had achieved registration by February 1992, but the number is now increasing at an exponential rate.

ISO and the ISO 9000 Series of Standards

The International Organization for Standardization, commonly referred to as "ISO," is a Geneva, Switzerland–based organization founded in 1946. It consists of 91 member countries and has approximately 180 technical committees whose mission is to develop and promote common standards (manufacturing, trade, and communication) worldwide to foster interactions and exchange of goods and services. The American National Standards Institute (ANSI) is the U.S. representative to ISO. The ISO 9000 series consists of five standards.[2]

ISO 9000

This document provides general standards for quality management and quality assurance and generic guidelines for the selection and application of ISO 9001, ISO 9002, and ISO 9003. It also provides guidelines for the use of ISO 9001 for the development, supply, and maintenance of software, as well as guidelines for the application of dependability management.

Futurescope

For many companies, especially those involved in international sales, achieving ISO registration is a necessity to compete in the marketplace of the 21st century. Likewise, many U.S. companies are now finding ISO 9000 to be a discriminating factor not only for foreign market entry, but also for landing domestic contracts. Today, the bottom line on global competitiveness is *quality,* regardless of whether a company is doing business in Europe, the Far East, or in the United States.

ISO 9001

The ISO 9001 standard provides a model of a quality assurance system for companies involved in the design, development, production, installation, and servicing of a product. This standard contains 20 clauses and is the standard most widely followed by industrial manufacturing companies.

ISO 9002

The ISO 9002 standard provides a model of a quality assurance system for companies involved in production, installation, and servicing but not involved in the design and development of a product. The standard contains 19 requirement clauses and is particularly relevant to the process industries (such as foundry, chemical, and food), manufacturers with standard product lines, or those engaged in production for original equipment manufacturers according to their specifications.

ISO 9003

The ISO 9003 standard, consisting of 16 requirement clauses, is a model of a quality assurance system for companies involved primarily in final inspection and testing. The standard typically applies to test houses, distributors, value-added contractors, and divisions within an organization.

ISO 9004

This document provides guidelines addressing the elements of quality management and quality assurance systems. In particular, it provides guidelines for services, processing material, quality improvement, and the application of the various elements of a quality management system.

The ISO 9000 series of standards is not a set of product standards, nor does the series regulate industry-specific criteria (such as automobile wheel diameters or the maximum chemical dosage in medicines). Rather, the standards provide a generic structure and requirements for establishing and maintaining a basic quality system to assure customers that the supplier company has the capability and systems to produce and provide quality products and/or services on time. Listed below are the headings of the 20 clauses comprising the ISO 9001 Standard:

1. Management Responsibility
2. Quality System (Principles)
3. Contract Review
4. Design Control
5. Document Control
6. Purchasing
7. Customer Supplier Product
8. Product Identification and Traceability
9. Process Control

10. Inspection and Testing
11. Inspection, Measuring and Test Equip.
12. Inspection and Test Status
13. Control of Nonconforming Product
14. Corrective Action
15. Handling, Storage, Packaging and Delivery
16. Quality Records
17. Internal Quality Audits
18. Training
19. Servicing
20. Statistical Techniques

The ISO 9000 series of standards is also generic in nature, the premise being that quality system requirements are essentially the same for all kinds of product offerings supplied by an organization. Thus the challenge is to select, interpret, and apply the appropriate standards in a way that both meets the requirements for registration and still satisfies the cost and practicality issues of a company.

Organization and Structure of an ISO 9000 Quality Assurance System

Clause 4.2 of the ISO 9001, ISO 9002, and ISO 9003 standards states that a company "shall establish and maintain a documented quality system as a means of ensuring that their product (or service) conforms to specified requirements." The clause does not state requirements per se, addressing how the quality system should be structured and documented. However, the "quality pyramid" has become a commonly suggested and accepted approach. The quality pyramid provides a structure whereby documentation is divided into four levels or tiers, as shown in Figure 1.

Level 1 documentation is the quality system manual, which typically describes the company's policy, commitment to quality, and approach to meet customers' needs and expectations. It also addresses the documentation structure of the quality system, the company's organizational structure, and the responsibilities of company management for maintaining the quality system and meeting the requirements of the various clauses of the standard. Because the quality manual addresses the company's quality policy and approach in a broad and concise manner, the manual is typically not more than 30–40 pages in length.

Level 2 documentation consists of the quality system procedures used to specify **who** does **what, when** it is done, and **what documentation** is used to verify that the quality activity was executed as required. If necessary to ensure quality, the procedure should also specify where the activity is to be performed. Procedures thus describe the steps each person or department must follow to meet the

Figure 1   "Quality Pyramid" Structure for Quality System Documentation

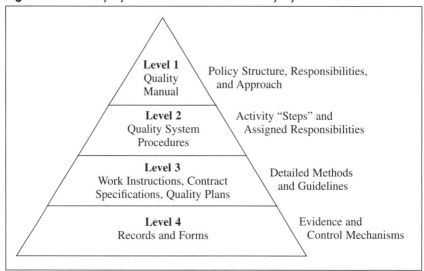

policies and responsibilities defined by the quality organization and approaches in the Level 1 quality manual.

Level 3 of the quality pyramid contains the work instructions used to specify **how** particular tasks are to be performed. Work instructions provide knowledge for decision making and/or guidelines addressing how to perform specific tasks. Work instructions thus provide detailed methods and guidelines in the form of instructions, checklists, diagrams, drawings, specifications, quality plans, and so forth. They are used to specify how particular tasks are to be performed and are required where the absence of such instructions would adversely affect quality.

Level 4 of the quality pyramid contains the records and forms used in the quality assurance system. Records are used to provide evidence that the required product or service quality was achieved, or to assure that the company's quality system has been implemented and adhered to correctly. Forms refer to the multitude of tags, labels, stickers, preprinted sheets, stamps, and other means to identify the status of materials, products, equipment, gauges, and devices used in the company to achieve the specified requirements.

In developing the documentation structure, it is important that the documentation across the four levels of the pyramid be interrelated and cross-referenced.

Documentation Development

The amount of documentation necessary to achieve registration depends on the type and size of the company. Although the standard does clearly specify where procedures are required, it is also clear that the standard does not state that all activities shall be documented. If not specified, system elements and activities must be documented only to the degree necessary to ensure adequate control. The extent of documentation required depends on the job skills needed, the degree of training acquired by the personnel involved in performing the activity, the size of the organization, the complexity of the quality system, the number of unskilled or part-time employees, and other factors that could adversely affect quality. A major challenge in implementation is thus to decide the appropriate level of documentation, considering both the requirements of the standard and the value of the documentation for providing adequate control and improving the consistency and quality of process operations.

Many companies currently reduce the time, effort, and expense in developing their quality system documentation by starting with generic manuals and procedures, often commercially available with a diskette for quick computer updating.[3] For example, although the company's quality manual must reflect its individual policy and commitment to quality, the nature and direct tie to the ISO standard makes it possible and efficient to generate the manual without "reinventing the wheel." A generic manual provides the general format and structure through which a company's management implementation team incorporates the unique aspects of the company's policy, commitment, and approach to quality. The management implementation team thus focuses on the important policy issues, organizational structures, and primary responsibilities necessary to establish and maintain an effective quality system.

Generic quality procedures are also commercially available in print and on diskette and provide a model of the content and format required in the procedure. Such generic procedures are often used by the procedure documentation development team to develop "personalized procedures" that can then be communicated to and approved by all appropriate personnel. This approach typically requires around 20–30 percent of the time needed to write a procedure from scratch.

Implementation: Steps, Costs, and Benefits

Achieving registration to ISO 9001, ISO 9002, or ISO 9003 is neither an easy nor an inexpensive task. Figure 2 lists the ten steps typically followed by a company in order to achieve registration. The average time to achieve ISO 9001 registration for medium-sized companies (fewer than 500 people) starting with a marginally structured quality assurance system is around 12–16 months. Costs for this same company can range from $20,000 to $40,000, which includes only expenses paid to the third-party registrar, not internal preparation and implementation costs. Such internal costs vary tremendously among organizations, depending on the complexity of their products and processes, the conformance level of their current quality system, and the implementation approach taken, to name just

Figure 2   Steps to Becoming Registered

1. Set up a steering group and define company objectives and scope of ISO 9000.

2. Evaluate current quality systems, reviewing existing procedures against ISO 9000 requirements.

3. Identify what needs to be done to bring the quality system into compliance and establish a program schedule and action plan.

4. Prepare/revise quality manual (policy, organization, responsibilities).

5. Select a registration agency and submit manual for approval (ASAP).

6. Prepare/revise operating procedures and work instructions, provide training, and implement new procedures.

7. Perform internal quality audits, checking compliance and quality audit system effectiveness, and institute corrective action on nonconformances found.

8. Perform precertification audit and institute corrective action on nonconformances found (optional).

9. Have official third-party registrar perform compliance audit/assessment and institute corrective action on nonconformances found.

10. Receive registration certificate upon follow-up (if required) and verification of successful completion of corrective action.

a few of the relevant factors. A rough estimate of internal costs for a company as described above is anywhere from $50,000 to $250,000.

In a recent survey of registered company executives in the United Kingdom, conducted by SGS Yarsley Quality Assured Firms, 50 percent of registered companies claimed to have recouped the cost of registration along with the consulting fees within three years of registration; 10 percent in less than two years; and 30 percent in 30 months.[4]

Although following the ten steps to become registered can be time-consuming and costly, the benefits are usually well worth the investment. A recent study in the United Kingdom found that ISO 9000–registered companies are reporting savings equal to 5 percent of total sales during the first two years after registration.[5] The survey, which included 2,317 registered companies with fewer than 500 employees across the industry sectors, also showed the following:

- 89 percent reported greater operational efficiency.
- 76 percent reported an improvement in marketing.
- 48 percent reported increased profitability.
- 26 percent reported increased export sales.

In general, registered companies experience a competitive advantage over those not registered, not only in the European community and other foreign markets, but domestically as well. As with all new strategies or technologies, the competitive advantage will be short-lived as ISO 9000–registered quality systems will become the norm and a minimum requirement for doing business. W. Edwards Deming is often quoted on his sarcastic statement, "You don't have to do this—survival is not compulsory!" For those companies wishing to establish and maintain a competitive marketing position, ISO 9000 is often a necessity.

References

1. Durand, Ian G., Donald W. Marquardt, Robert W. Peach, and James C. Pyle, Updating the ISO 9000 Quality Standards: Responding to Marketplace Needs," *Quality Progress* (July 1993).

2. The ISO 9000 series of standards was adopted word for word by the United States as the ANSI/ASQC Q90 series of standards. (ANSI is the American National Standards Institute and ASQC is the American Society for Quality Control.)

3. Steudel, Harold J., *ISO 9001 Sample Quality Manual* (Madison, Wisc.: H.J. Steudel & Associates, Inc., 1992).

4. *Quality Systems Update* (Fairfax, Va.: CEEM Publications, February 1993).

5. *Survey of Quality Consultancy Scheme Clients 1988–90* (United Kingdom: Pera International and Salford University Business Services Limited, September 1991).

—49—
ZERO-DEFECT
MARKETING
SYSTEMS

Allan J. Magrath

Allan J. Magrath is a full-time marketing executive and part-time marketing educator, author, and consultant. He holds an H.B.A. and M.B.A. from Western's Business School. He is Director of Marketing Services and New Business Ventures for 3M Canada, where he manages marketing research, strategic planning, marketing training, creative services, and new business ventures for the company. He has published more than 100 articles in 25 major journals. He is the author of *The Six Imperatives of Marketing* and *How to Achieve Zero-Defect Marketing*.

PepsiCo Inc. took a look at its marketing channel system and decided it needed an overhaul. So now, consumers can find Pizza Hut, Taco Bell, and Kentucky Fried Chicken offerings inside 650 of the nation's supermarkets in addition to their 22,000-plus restaurant sites. Gillette examined its product innovation system and found it lacked the focus and tactical control necessary to roll out a global "hit" product. So they centralized the marketing for the Sensor razor program in Boston, reducing the power of local brand managers around the world in areas such as advertising, promotions, and product positioning. The result was a much more polished, coherent, and successful new-product launch.

United Parcel Service (UPS) put its marketing planning and research system under the microscope and discovered high customer dissatisfaction with its inflexible pricing and service, as well as an inappropriate concentration on home deliveries versus corporate business. UPS invested heavily in focus-group research with customers, beefed up its corporate business marketing, and became price-competitive. As a result, its revenues and profits are growing faster than their rivals', and customer satisfaction has increased significantly. All of these examples point to corporations that have reengineered one or another of their fundamental systems in marketing for added growth or margin improvement. Having mapped their marketing processes, PepsiCo, Gillette, and UPS were able to spot holes in their approaches and change these selected processes for the better.

Marketing Systems

Although system or process mapping is commonplace in manufacturing, logistics, and administration, it is not as common or well understood in marketing. Marketing has tended to be program-oriented around the model of the marketing mix, involving pricing, product, promotion, and place (distribution). In fact, marketing

Futurescope

Marketers are often tuned into tasks and programs, rather than systems thinking. Yet by mapping marketing systems, it is possible to greatly improve their characteristics or outputs, from yield to cycle time to waste minimization. In the 21st century, marketing will experience as much pressure as the factory to improve productivity. Zero-defect principles applied to marketing's processes offer the promise of reengineering systems for the benefit of both the firm's customers and its own sales and marketing work force.

Figure 1   The Multiple Systems of Marketing

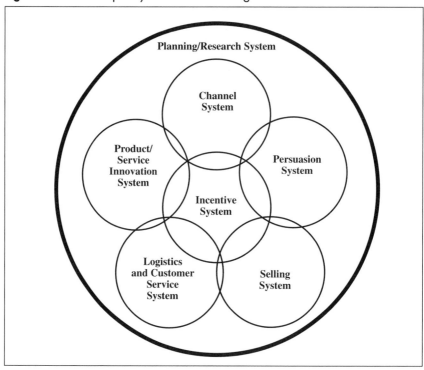

is the sum total of seven major systems, each of which can be mapped. These systems are:

1. The planning/research system

2. The product/service innovation system

3. The selling system

4. The channel system

5. The persuasion system

6. The incentive system

7. The logistics and customer service system

Each system is linked to the others, and each involves components that can be mapped in sequence. Figure 1 illustrates these seven connected systems.

Mapping Components
of a Marketing System

Figure 2 outlines what components are involved in a typical selling system. On the left are those components managed by sales reps, for instance, their customer records, available sales time, self-development, and so forth. On the right side of the diagram and connected to reps are sales managers, with components they control and emphasize (such as deploying reps, compensation planning, training, etc.).

By breaking a system apart, it is possible to examine which components are working well and which are not, according to factors generally associated with TQM (total quality management) practice. These include criteria such as costs, waste, flexibility, yield, cycle time, and other issues. In general, these can be termed zero-defect marketing issues, because they emphasize the system's results on a broader array of measurements than macromeasures such as growth or market share.

Figure 2   The Selling System's Two Main Components and Their Functions

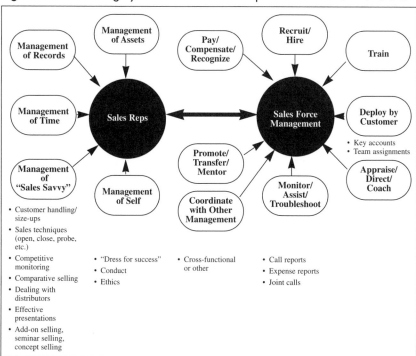

Source: Magrath, *How to Achieve Zero-Defect Marketing.*

Figure 3 shows how the application of zero-defect thinking could be applied to a selling system. Improvements in such TQM measures of a selling system translate into less waste, more flexibility, lower costs, and higher yields from a company's reps and sales managers. As Figure 3 illustrates, different possible system improvements are tied to which component of the system is in the greatest need of reengineering. If lowering the system's costs is the critical issue, solutions can

Figure 3. Initiatives for Total Quality Sales Force Management

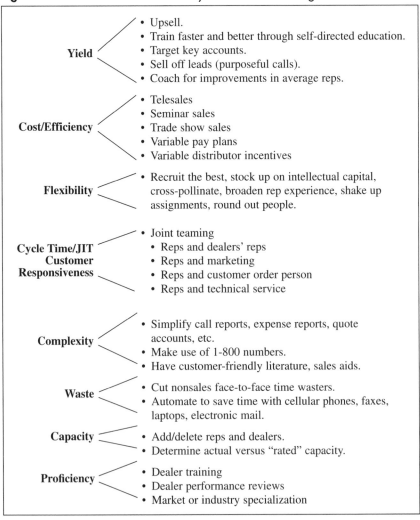

Yield
- Upsell.
- Train faster and better through self-directed education.
- Target key accounts.
- Sell off leads (purposeful calls).
- Coach for improvements in average reps.

Cost/Efficiency
- Telesales
- Seminar sales
- Trade show sales
- Variable pay plans
- Variable distributor incentives

Flexibility
- Recruit the best, stock up on intellectual capital, cross-pollinate, broaden rep experience, shake up assignments, round out people.

Cycle Time/JIT Customer Responsiveness
- Joint teaming
- Reps and dealers' reps
- Reps and marketing
- Reps and customer order person
- Reps and technical service

Complexity
- Simplify call reports, expense reports, quote accounts, etc.
- Make use of 1-800 numbers.
- Have customer-friendly literature, sales aids.

Waste
- Cut nonsales face-to-face time wasters.
- Automate to save time with cellular phones, faxes, laptops, electronic mail.

Capacity
- Add/delete reps and dealers.
- Determine actual versus "rated" capacity.

Proficiency
- Dealer training
- Dealer performance reviews
- Market or industry specialization

Source: Magrath, *How to Achieve Zero-Defect Marketing*

lie in lower-cost sales methods (telesales, seminar sales to sell customers in groups, variable pay plans that reward only if sales improve, etc.). If cycle time is the issue, different tactics are implemented, such as more teamwork with dealers or more contact between the sales force and other departments, such as customer service, the technical function, or marketing.

Figure 4.   Process Variables That Count in a Persuasion System

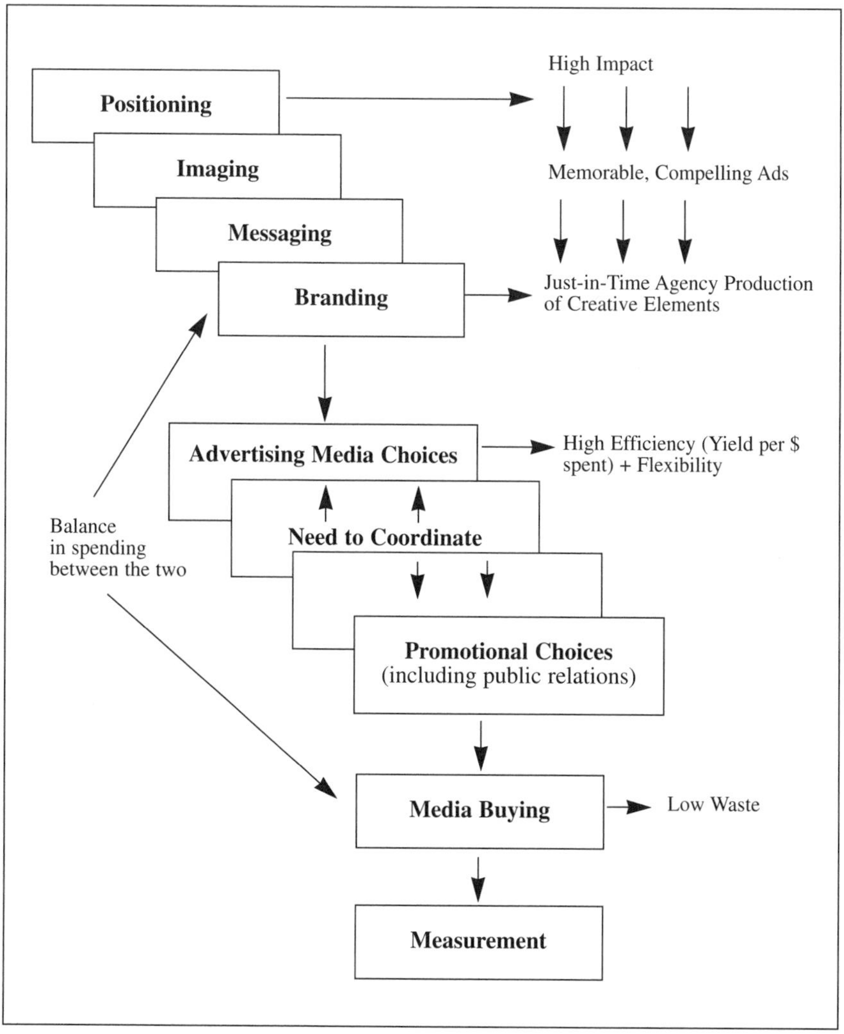

Source: Magrath, *How to Achieve Zero-Defect Marketing.*

Figure 5 Creative Yield Methods

- Recycling (RCA, Timex, Old Spice)
- Extensions
- Families versus one-up brands (cross-selling)
- Consistency in theming (Maytag, Michelin, Heinz, Fed Ex)
- Cross-promotions
- Variable commissions with agencies
- Corporation-identity policy—coordinate all of its various facets, including print, electronic, point of sale, and packaging graphic images
- Modularity of creative work for use in multiple media

Source: Magrath, *How to Achieve Zero-Defect Marketing.*

Deciding Which Marketing System to Fix

Using a zero-defect mindset and applying it to one of the seven marketing systems calls for a compass. Otherwise, the firm would try to improve all of its systems and various components at once, losing the speed and leverage that would accompany focusing on the system that is most critical to adding value from the customer's perspective.

For example, a consumer giant such as Nestle or Philip Morris might hone in on its persuasion system for the highest payback from a TQM approach, because

Figure 6. Media Waste Minimization

- Buy bundled deals or sell-offs
- Avoid competitor clutter
- Niche where possible for high specificity by selecting
  - Regional versus national media
  - Direct mail versus print
  - Trade shows versus journals
  - Specialty magazines versus general print media
  - New networks such as MTV, senior channels, Whittle in schools
  - Videocassettes to home
- Coordinate with PR, promotions
- Piggybacking on events

Source: Magrath, *How to Achieve Zero-Defect Marketing.*

persuasion is the key system that builds the equity of its brands and thereby the confidence consumers place in these brands. A computer company such as Apple, Compaq, or IBM might prioritize its channel system as a key lever to influence market share and presence.

Figure 4 diagrams a typical marketing persuasion system. Applying zero-defect thinking could result in suggested improvements to the front-end "creative" development part of the system or the media selection/buying component of the system. Figures 5 and 6 show how these two components might be improved.

Mapping a firm's processes or systems is not new. Used extensively in manufacturing, logistics, and administrative areas, process mapping is a rich vein to mine for improved performance. By mapping systems in any company, bottlenecks can be spotted and costs of various activity steps identified. Process mapping provides a way of visualizing where time delays and costs pile up needlessly. And from this assessment can come ideas to alter the system fundamentally and cut both costs and activity cycle times, which translates into customer benefits.

–50–

BENCHMARKING

C. Jackson Grayson, Jr.

C. Jackson Grayson, Jr., is founder and chairman of the Houston-based American Productivity & Quality Center. The Center is a nonprofit business education, training, and research organization dedicated to improving productivity, quality, and quality of work life. Grayson was instrumental in the founding of the International Benchmarking Clearinghouse, the Center's full-service benchmarking operation.

Benchmarking is one of the new terms streaking across the management skies. Some people think it's a fad and that it has nothing to do with productivity and quality. They're wrong.

It's a continuous comparison of your processes with the best (domestic and foreign) from inside and outside your industry. *Benchmarking* has become a common term since it was popularized by Xerox in the 1980s. It has become recognized as an essential ingredient in the success of Malcolm Baldridge National Quality Award winners. Perhaps the simplest way to introduce benchmarking is to answer some of the common questions people have about this concept.

What Is a Benchmark?

There is a distinction between the word *benchmark* and the process of benchmarking. The word *benchmark* comes from geographic surveying, in which it means to take a measurement against a reference point. In the quality improvement lexicon, a benchmark is a "best-in-class" achievement. This achievement then becomes the reference point or recognized standard of excellence against which similar processes are measured.

What Is the Process of Benchmarking?

Whereas a benchmark is a measure, benchmarking is a process of measurement. It is a business process that can contribute to achieving competitive advantage. During the creation of the International Benchmarking Clearinghouse (the newest division of the American Productivity & Quality Center), the members of the design steering committee developed a working definition of benchmarking:

Futurescope

Best practices know no border of political, industrial, or geographic dimensions. They can be found in Europe, Japan, or North America; in health care, manufacturing, government, or educational organizations; in democratic, nationalistic, or dictatorial nations. As we approach the 21st century, the economic borders of the world are shrinking, and the need for competitive awareness on a global perspective has increased. Benchmarking recognizes that the improvement of quality and productivity is a win-win situation for every member country of the world's economic community.

Benchmarking is the process of continuously comparing and measuring an organization with business leaders anywhere in the world to gain information which will help the organization take action to improve its performance.

Benchmarking is an ongoing measurement and analysis process that compares practices, processes, or methodologies to those of other organizations. The purpose of these studies is to identify best practices that can be adapted to a wide range of organizations and to provide them with quantum process improvements, which result in increased business performance.

While there are many ways to benchmark, there are two distinct approaches: competitive benchmarking and process benchmarking.

1. **Competitive benchmarking** measures organizational performance against that of competing organizations. Competitive benchmarking tends to concentrate on the relative performance of competitors using a select set of measures.

2. **Process benchmarking** measures discrete process performance and functionality against organizations that lead in those processes. Process benchmarking seeks the best practice for conducting a particular business process after first validating that the performance of that process is, indeed, world-class. Once the best practice is identified and understood, then it can be adapted and improved for application to another organization.

What Benchmarking Is **Not**

It might be helpful to define the process of benchmarking by explaining what benchmarking is *not*. Benchmarking is not competitive analysis. Competitive analysis is a comparison of yourself to competitors in your industry, largely in macro terms of market share, financial measures, etc. Although it is useful for planning broad strategy, competitive analysis does not go to the next level required for process improvement.

Benchmarking is also not a copying procedure, although it does involve observing and learning about the best practices of others. If you carbon-copy their practices, that is copying. But that rarely works. Things are seldom exactly the same between firms, i.e., in structure or resources, so you must adapt their methods to fit yours.

The process is not just numbers, like comparisons in terms of time, cost, and quality. Such numerical comparisons are useful in calibrating the size of the gap, but it is much more important to discover how they arrived at those numbers.

Benchmarking is not restricted to manufacturing. Facets of your organization are candidates for the procedure. In the same vein, it applies equally to education, health care, defense, and government.

As a cooperative mechanism, it cannot open every door, because organizations don't share their most competitive secrets. But that leaves a very large number of processes that competitors will share, as has already been proven. Compaq and Apple, for example, have benchmarked certain processes with each other.

Who is Benchmarked?

Perhaps the most difficult aspect of a benchmarking study is identifying the appropriate target companies or benchmarking partners. The various classes of companies to be benchmarked were described earlier: internal, competitive, industry or functional, and generic. The key question is how do you identify which particular company should receive the detailed attention of a benchmarking study? The primary tool used to answer this question is secondary research. This is the process of identifying, through literature search and personal contacts, which companies perform the process in an exceptional manner. Industry award winners, functional excellence recognition, and national quality award presentations are three indicators of excellence that help to separate one company from another. However, the truly excellent company might not choose to apply or compete for an award. That company might not want its process excellence to be displayed for all to see. Building a network of personal contacts can lead to the richest sources of organizations to benchmark.

A word of caution is needed. Gaining access at the appropriate level is a critical success factor in conducting benchmarking studies. Some companies that are known for excellent processes, for example, L.L. Bean, Xerox, or Federal Express, have been inundated with requests for benchmarking on the same topic by a variety of companies. These companies have a need to reduce the redundancy in the replies, while maintaining a responsive attitude to requests from companies that might be their customers or suppliers. The winners of the Malcolm Baldridge National Quality Award know that they have not achieved "best-in-class" status on every one of their business processes. However, many companies make the mistake of believing that their target benchmarking partner should be a company that has been awarded the Baldridge Award.

Selecting the right company and finding the right contact within that company are two of the most troublesome areas for new benchmarkers. Those who are experienced in benchmarking have built their personal network of contacts and work their list to gain access to the process owners within the targeted benchmark partner company.

How Is a Benchmarking Study Completed?

Benchmarking studies can take many forms: telephone surveys, written questionnaires, literature searches, exchange of prepared materials, or site visits. Benchmarking studies generally follow a four-step process: planning a benchmarking project, collecting data, analyzing the data for performance gaps and process enablers, and improving by adapting process enablers.

What Is the Result of a Benchmarking Study?

A benchmarking study can provide outputs. First, it should provide a measure that compares performance for the benchmarked process among the target organizations. Second, it should describe the organization's gap in performance as compared to these identified performance levels. Third, it should identify best practices and enablers that produced the results observed during the study. Finally, the study should set performance goals for the process and identify areas where action can be taken to improve the sponsoring organization's performance. The sponsoring organization is then responsible for implementing the action plan.

How Have Benchmarking Studies Influenced Organizations?

Benchmarking studies have been used to position companies strategically. Xerox uses benchmarking information to set goals for its principle measures of business performance and has reported significant savings as a result of applying the results of benchmarking studies. Other organizations that have obtained significant successes from benchmarking include Alcoa, AT&T, Digital Equipment Corporation, DuPont, Hewlett-Packard, IBM, Johnson & Johnson, Kodak, Milliken, Motorola, Texas Instruments, Westinghouse, and Weyerhaeuser. In these cases, the benefit derived from benchmarking is threefold:

1. Building awareness of the best practice for performance in a particular process

2. Learning the measure of excellence for the targeted process

3. Applying these lessons within the sponsoring organization where they can be used to improve performance results.

It is not uncommon to achieve savings in the hundreds of thousands of dollars as a result of applying the benchmarking process for continuous improvement. The ratio of results to costs for benchmarking studies can be greater than five to one.

An International Clearinghouse for Benchmarking

A clearinghouse is needed to help foster the use of benchmarking and facilitate the sharing of information and techniques among a wider audience of organizations. The vision for the International Benchmarking Clearinghouse is to provide leadership in promoting, facilitating, and improving benchmarking to improve quality and productivity in organizations throughout the world. Although the clearinghouse is based in the United States and seeks to improve the competitiveness of American organizations, it is also international, providing services and promoting the use of benchmarking worldwide.

About the
Contributors

Doug Adams is president of the Efficient Consumer Response (ECR) and Operational Applications Division of Nielsen Marketing Research NA. As such, he is responsible for developing and directing the company's ECR activities, including designing and implementing strategies and tactics, products and services, and marketing. He is also responsible for several specific product areas, including coordinating daily store-level data acquisition and processing, ECR software applications, and logistic management systems. Adams has been a regular speaker at industry conferences in the United States and Europe. He holds a bachelor's degree in economics and an M.B.A. in finance and marketing from Emory University.

Tony Alessandra, Ph.D., is a leading sales speaker and trainer based in La Jolla, California. He has authored numerous books, audio, and video programs, including *Collaborative Selling, Idea-A-Day Guide to Super Selling,* and *The Competitive Advantage.*

Richard G. Barlow is Founder and President of Frequency Marketing Inc., a marketing agency specializing in the development and implementation of marketing programs aimed at improving customer retention and enhancing share of customer. He is also the publisher of *COLLOQUY,* a quarterly frequency marketing journal produced by Frequency Marketing Inc.

Greg Baron is a Certified Management Consultant with extensive experience in the areas of customer service, team building, sales development, collaboration, executive coaching, and Neuro Linguistic Programming (NLP). As Founder and

President of Success Sciences, he has developed his expertise through working with a wide variety of organizations including Motorola, USA Today, Florida Power, Sony, Pioneer, IBM, Continental Airlines, and Novell. He is the author of *The Idea-A-Day Guide to Super Selling* and *Customer Service,* as well as numerous articles in professional journals.

Rena Bartos is President of the Rena Bartos Company. A consultant and writer, she counsels on communications and consumer issues, and is the author of *Marketing to Women Around the World, The Moving Target: What Every Marketer Should Know About Women, Advertising and Consumers—New Perspectives, The Future of the Advertising Agency Research Function,* and *The Founding Fathers of Advertising Research.* She was formerly a Senior Vice President and Director of Communications Development at the J. Walter Thompson Company. She holds degrees from Rutgers University and Columbia University.

Harold A. Bergen is Executive Vice President of Ruder-Finn, Chicago. He served companies, associations, and governments in corporate, financial, marketing, employee, government, crisis management, and community relations programs. Before entering public relations, he was an editor of *Industry and Power* magazine, senior associate editor of *Consulting Engineer* magazine, and manager of technical publications for the Raytheon Company. He is an active member of the Public Relations Society of America, and has written and lectured extensively on public relations.

Kate Bertrand is a freelance writer based in Pacifica, California. Former editor of *Software Marketing Journal* and former West Coast editor of *Business Marketing,* Ms. Bertrand has written for *Advertising Age, Marketing Computers, British Business,* and many other business and consumer publications. She co-authored *Developing a Winning JIT Marketing Strategy* with Charles O'Neal, and has contributed to textbooks on marketing, advertising, and biology.

Ken Bieschke is President of Aggressive List Management, Inc., a full-service list and P.I.P. marketing/management firm dealing exclusively in areas related to the creation, maintenance, marketing, fulfillment, and accounting support of mailing list rental and package insert programs. He holds a B.B.A. degree from the University of Notre Dame and an M.B.A. from Northwestern Graduate School of Management, both in marketing.

Frank V. Cespedes received his B.A. from the City College of New York, his M.S. from the Massachusetts Institute of Technology, and his Ph.D. from Cornell University. For fifteen years, he has been a faculty member at Harvard Business School, where he has taught in various M.B.A. and Executive Education programs. He is also a faculty partner at The Center for Executive Development in Cambridge, Massachusetts. He is the author of *Concurrent Marketing: Managing Product, Sales, and Service Linkages; Organizing and Implementing the Marketing Effort; Going to Market: Distribution Systems for Industrial Products;* as well as articles in *Harvard Business Review, California Management Review, Industrial Marketing, Marketing Research, Organization Science, Journal of Consumer Marketing, Journal of Marketing Channels, Sloan Management Review,* and other journals.

Larry Chiagouris is Executive Vice President, Director of Client and Strategic Services, Creamer Dickson Basford Public Relations and founder of BrandMarketing Services, Ltd., a strategic marketing and research consulting company. He has served on the board of directors of the American Marketing Association and the Advertising Research Foundation and has counseled many leading packaged goods, services and technology companies, to include AT&T, General Foods, Panasonic, Citibank and Pfizer. He holds a Ph.D. from CUNY in Marketing and a B.S. in Economics from New York University.

Richard J. Chvala serves as an adjunct professor at the University of Richmond School of Business Management. He is Senior Consultant, Sales and Marketing Training, for Ethyl Corporation, a Fortune 500 company based in Richmond, Virginia. Chvala also serves on the national board of the American Marketing Association, and was the keynote speaker at the AMA's First International Congress on Customer Satisfaction. Rich has more than 15 years of experience as a national sales manager and marketing executive for both capital goods and service companies. Chvala's training specialties include strategic selling, customer communications, and creating value for the customer. He is the co-author of *Total Quality and Marketing.* Chvala received his undergraduate degree in biochemistry from Michigan Technological University and his M.B.A. from Michigan.

Philip B. Crosby worked for 27 years as a quality management professional for Martin Marietta and ITT. He is the author of *Cutting the Cost of Quality, Quality Is Free,* and *Completeness: Quality for the 21st Century.* He is featured in a weekly commentary, "On Improvement," on USA News' "First Business" television program.

Michael R. Czinkota, Ph.D., is one of the nation's top international business and marketing experts. Serving as Deputy Assistant Secretary of Commerce during the Reagan Administration, Dr. Czinkota continues to advise government bodies and corporations on international trade, financing, and investment. A faculty member at Georgetown University, Dr. Czinkota publishes and is interviewed extensively in the trade press. He is a frequent and dynamic speaker on international issues.

Bob Donath is a well-known speaker and author on the subjects of business-to-business advertising and marketing. His career represents a unique combination of experience and accomplishment in the fields of publishing, journalism, and marketing management. Mr. Donath now heads his own marketing and marketing communications consulting firm, Bob Donath & Co., in White Plains, New York, specializing in business-to-business marketing. His clients include marketing services firms, corporate marketing communications departments, and a business-academic think tank at a major university. He is the author of *Managing Sales Leads: How to Turn Every Prospect into a Customer,* and is a regularly featured columnist in the American Marketing Association's *Marketing News* newspaper. Mr. Donath holds a master's degree in marketing from Northwestern University's Kellogg School of Management, and a bachelor's degree from Northwestern's Medill School of Journalism.

Adel I. El-Ansary is the Eminent Scholar and first chairholder of the Paper and Plastics Education and Research (PAPER) Foundation Endowed Research Chair in Wholesaling at the College of Business Administration of the University of North Florida. In addition to his duties as Research Professor, he serves as Director of the Center for Research and Education in Wholesaling. He holds a Bachelor of Commerce degree from Cairo University, Cairo, Egypt, and an M.B.A. and Ph.D. from Ohio State University, Columbus, Ohio.

O.C. Ferrell is Interim Dean and Distinguished Professor of Marketing and Business Ethics in the Fogelman College of Business and Economics at The University of Memphis. Dr. Ferrell was chairman of the American Marketing Association Ethics Committee that developed the current AMA Code of Ethics. He has published articles on marketing ethics in the *Journal of Marketing, Journal of Marketing Research, Journal of Business Research, Journal of Macromarketing, Journal of the Academy of Marketing Science, Journal of Advertising, Human Relations, Journal of Business Ethics,* as well as others. He has co-authored ten textbooks including a leading basic marketing text, *Marketing: Concepts and Strategies,* Ninth Edition, and *Business Ethics: Ethical Decision Making and Cases,* Second Edition, and a tradebook, *In Pursuit of Ethics.*

Shaun P. Gilmore is Vice President of Global Consumer Communications Services for AT&T. He has held a variety of management positions at AT&T since first arriving at the firm in 1980, including both Operations Vice President of Inbound Services and Director of 800 Services Product Management and Marketing. He holds an M.B.A. in finance from Harvard Business School.

Greg Goodman, EdD, is Process Manager of the All-Employee Systems Division of Maritz, Inc., a performance improvement firm based in Fenton, Missouri. Since joining Maritz, Goodman has worked with such clients as Siemens Medical Systems, IDS, General American Life, McDonald's, AT&T, Mallinckrodt

Medical, General Electric, Ameritech, Georgia-Pacific, Transamerica, Bristol Mey-ers-Squibb, Baylor Medical Center, Monsanto, General Motors, and Fort Sanders Health System. He holds a doctorate degree in education from the University of Massachusetts-Amherst; an M.A. in biomedical communications from The Ohio State University; and a B.S., summa cum laude, in broadcasting, also from The Ohio State University.

C. Jackson Grayson, Jr., is founder and chairman of the Houston-based Ameri-can Productivity & Quality Center. The Center is a nonprofit business education, training, and research organization dedicated to improving productivity, quality, and quality of work life. Grayson was instrumental in the founding of the Inter-national Benchmarking Clearinghouse, the Center's full-service benchmarking operation.

John R. Hauser is the Kirin Professor of Marketing at Massachusetts Institute of Technology's Sloan School of Management. He is the head of Sloan's Marketing Group, co-director of Sloan's International Center for Research on the Manage-ment of Technology, and Editor-in-Chief of *Marketing Science.* Dr. Hauser is the co-author of two textbooks, *Design and Marketing of New Products* and *Essen-tials of New Product Management,* and two computer-based texts/software pack-ages, *Applying Marketing Management* and *Enterprise: An Integrating Man-agement Exercise,* and has published more than 40 scientific articles. In addition to writing, teaching, and researching, Dr. Hauser has also served as a consultant to leading corporations in many industries.

Michael Herrington is a consultant in Total Quality Management and business process redesign, and is located in Fairfield, Connecticut. He has worked with numerous clients in the development and implementation of their quality improve-ment strategies. Using both the Malcolm Baldridge National Quality Award cri-teria and the criteria for the Connecticut Award for Excellence, he has led organizational assessments and subsequent implementation of organization qual-ity improvement initiatives. Prior to entering consulting, Herrington was Vice Pres-ident for Quality Improvement for Olin Corporation. He is a graduate of The Ohio State University, and holds a degree in mechanical engineering.

Cecil C. Hoge, Sr. is Chairman of Harrison-Hoge Industries, Inc. and of Huber Hoge & Sons Advertising, Inc. He is the author of *Mail Order Moonlighting, Mail Order Know-How, What We Can Learn from the Century of Competition Between Sears and Wards: The first 100 Years Are the Toughest,* and *The Electronic Mar-keting Manual,* as well as countless shorter pieces and works-in-progress. He has been interviewed on over 1,000 radio and television stations, in various publica-tions, and on line, and has lectured extensively, as well.

Philip Kotler is the S.C. Johnson & Son Distinguished Professor of International Marketing at Northwestern University's J.L. Kellogg Graduate School of Management. He is the author of more than 100 articles and 15 books, including *Marketing Management; Strategic Marketing for Nonprofit Organizations; Social Marketing; Marketing Places; Marketing Models;* and *The New Competition.* He has been a consultant to such companies as IBM, General Electric, AT&T, Bank of America, Merck, Motorola, Ford, and others. He holds honorary degrees from the University of Zurich and DePaul University, and has been a director or board of advisors member of the American Marketing Association, Marketing Science Institute, The Drucker Foundation, Gemini, and The School of the Art Institute of Chicago. He received his M.A. from the University of Chicago and his Ph.D. from Massachusetts Institute of Technology, both in economics.

Alan K. Leahigh is Executive Vice President of Public Communications Inc., counselors in corporate, marketing, public affairs, financial, and institutional communications. A partner in the firm, he has more than 25 years of professional communications experience, and shares management responsibility for marketing, public affairs, health care, and general public relations accounts. He holds a bachelor of arts degree in political science from Illinois Wesleyan University, Bloomington, and a master of arts in journalism from the University of Missouri, Columbia.

J. Raymond Lewis, Jr. joined Holiday Inn Worldwide in 1985, after nearly two decades of experience in sales, marketing, and advertising. He is currently Executive Vice President of Worldwide Sales & Marketing. Lewis is a member of the board and executive committee of Holiday Inn Worldwide, and is a member of the Association of National Advertisers and the National Advertising Review Board. He has also served on the Services Marketing Council of the American Marketing Association and is a member of the American Management Association. In addition, he has been active in a number of civic organizations.

Allan J. Magrath is a full-time marketing executive and part-time marketing educator, author, and consultant. He holds an H.B.A. and M.B.A. from the Business School of the University of Western Ontario. He is Director of Marketing Services and New Business Ventures for 3M Canada, where he manages marketing research, strategic planning, marketing training, creative services, and new business ventures for the company. He has published more than 100 articles in 25 major journals. He is the author of *The Six Imperatives of Marketing* and *How to Achieve Zero-Defect Marketing.*

Jeffrey W. Marr joined Indianapolis-based Walker Research in 1977 and is now Vice President, Client Services. He has ultimate responsibility for a variety of W:CSM (Walker Customer Service Management) national and multinational accounts. He holds a B.A. from Indiana University. He is a member of the American Marketing Association, the American Society for Quality Control, the Conference Board and the Marketing Science Institute.

Robert S. Menchin is a recognized authority on marketing to mature consumers. In a career spanning more than 25 years, he has written four books and hundreds of articles, brochures, booklets, ads, direct mail campaigns, newsletters, sales presentations, and seminar programs for Fortune 500 companies and other major international firms. As former Vice President of Member Relation and Communications of the Chicago Board of Trade (the oldest and largest futures exchange in the world) and head of Wall Street Marketing Communications (a Chicago-based consulting firm), he has an established following in the mature market network.

John T. Mentzer, Ph.D., is the Bruce Excellence Chair of Business Policy at the University of Tennessee Department of Marketing, Logistics, and Transportation, Knoxville. He has published in *Industrial Marketing Management, Journal of the Academy of Marketing Science, Columbia Journal of World Business, Research in Marketing, Journal of Business Logistics, International Journal of Physical Distribution and Logistics Management, Transportation and Logistics Review, Transportation Journal,* and other journals.

Gerald A. Michaelson is an experienced corporate executive who has worked for several Fortune 500 companies. He is Executive Vice President of Tennessee Associates International, a management consulting firm based in Knoxville, Tennessee. His book *Winning the Marketing War* has been acclaimed as the best book on strategy ever written.

Gary M. Mullet, Ph.D., is President and Principal of Gary Mullet Associates, Inc., a consulting and statistical data processing firm concentrating on marketing research. His work experience includes time with Sophisticated Data Research and Burke Marketing Research. He has taught at the Universities of Cincinnati and Michigan, and at Georgia Institute of Technology. He has published several articles on statistics and marketing research and is active in various professional organizations as a reviewer and a presenter. His degrees are from Central Michigan University, North Carolina State University, and the University of Michigan. His clients include both marketing research suppliers and end-users of research.

Jerry J. Neal is Manager of Marketing Program Management at the Public Service Company of New Mexico. He has more than 20 years of experience in the electric utility industry in the areas of customer service, marketing and sales, technical analysis of residential and commercial buildings, and electric utility system engineering analysis. Neal attended the University of New Mexico, where he earned an M.A. in management from the Robert O. Anderson Graduate School of

Management and a B.S. in electrical engineering. He was a founding member of the New Mexico chapter of the American Marketing Association, and later served as the chapter's second president. During his tenure as president, the chapter was named as Chapter of the Year. Neal also serves as a member of the AMA's Professional Chapters Council, and is the president and owner of a utility marketing consulting business, Prescriptive Services.

Jacqueline A. Ottman is the president of J. Ottman Consulting, Inc., a strategic resource that she founded in 1989 to advise forward-thinking companies on the development and promotion of environmentally sound products. Her clients include Colgate-Palmolive, Kraft General Foods, DuPont, General Electric, and Eastman-Kodak. A pioneer in environmental marketing, Ms. Ottman is the creator of the *Getting to Zero*SM process, the first concept-generation process specifically designed for environment-related new product invention. She is author of the award-winning book, *Green Marketing: Challenges and Opportunities for the New Marketing Age,* and a co-author of *Environmental Consumerism: What Every Marketer Needs to Know,* and *Green Marketing Anthology.* She also is a featured columnist for *American Marketplace* and *Marketing News,* and is a sought-after speaker at conferences in the United States and abroad.

Allan R. Paison is President and CEO of Walker: Customer Satisfaction Measurements. Prior to joining Walker in 1983, he worked for NFO Research and Xerox Corporation. Mr. Paison speaks regularly on the topic of customer satisfaction measurement in domestic and international marketing. He is on the Boards of Advisors of the First Interstate Center for Service Marketing (Arizona State University), the Institute for the Study of Business Markets (Penn State University), the Services Marketing Center (Vanderbilt University), and the Center for Customer-Driven Quality (Purdue University), and is Trustee of the Marketing Sciences Institute.

B. Joseph Pine II is the founder and President of Ridgefield, Connecticut-based Strategic Horizons, Inc., a management consulting firm specializing in helping companies envision and then realize their futures. Mr. Pine is the author of the highly acclaimed book *Mass Customization: The New Frontier in Business Competition,* which *The Financial Times* named one of the top business books of 1993. In it he details the historic shift from mass production to mass customization— the low-cost, high-quality creation of individually customized goods and services. He has also written articles for a number of magazines and journals, including the *Harvard Business Review, The Wall Street Journal, Planning Review,* the *IBM Systems Journal, Chief Executive,* and *CIO.*

Al Ries is chairman of Ries & Ries, a marketing strategy firm based in Great Neck, New York. Prior to establishing Ries & Ries, he was founder and chairman of the board of Trout & Ries, where he worked with Jack Trout for more than 26 years. Together, Trout and Ries have co-authored a number of industry classics and best-sellers, including *Positioning: The Battle for Your Mind; Marketing Warfare;* and *Bottom-Up Marketing.* Their latest book, *The 22 Immutable Laws of Marketing,* outlines the basic reasons marketing programs succeed or fail.

Howard Schlossberg is the author of a forthcoming book on sports marketing for Blackwell Publishers. He wrote a column on sports marketing for three years in the American Marketing Association's biweekly magazine, *Marketing News.* For the past 20 years, Schlossberg has covered prep athletics in the Chicago area, first for Pioneer Press and currently for Paddock Publications. His coverage has been recognized for excellence by the Northern Illinois Newspaper Association, the Sub-urban Newspaper of America, and the National Association of Softball Writers and Broadcasters. At 43, Schlossberg's work has appeared in everything from *Advertising Age* to *Restaurants & Institutions.* He also contributes to the hockey magazine *Blueline,* and is Chicago correspondent for the Sports Network wire service. He teaches journalism at William Rainey Harper College, and is currently at work on his second book.

Don E. Schultz, Ph.D., is a professor of Integrated Marketing Communications at the Medill School of Journalism at Northwestern University. In 1974, he gave up his position as Senior Vice President of Tracy-Locke Advertising and Public Relations to launch his career in academia. He obtained his master's degree in advertising and his Ph.D. in mass media from Michigan State University, and joined Northwestern in 1977. Schultz has written, consulted, held seminars, and lectured extensively on sales, marketing, advertising, and integrated marketing communications, is active in numerous professional organizations, and is President of Agora, Inc., a marketing, advertising, and consulting firm.

Michael V. Scherman is an engineering consultant at H.J. Steudel & Associates, Inc., where he is involved in training and implementing systems for quality and productivity improvement. He earned a B.S. degree in industrial engineering and an M.S. degree in manufacturing systems engineering from the University of Wisconsin–Madison.

Jagdish N. Sheth, Ph.D., is the Charles Kellstadt Professor of Marketing at Emory University. Formerly, he was the Robert Brooker Professor of Marketing at the University of Southern California and the Walter Stellner Distinguished Professor of Marketing at the University of Illinois. Dr. Sheth has published numerous books and articles in marketing and other business disciplines and has received numerous awards for his work, including the P.D. Converse Award from the American Marketing Association.

G. Lynn Shostack is Chairman, President, and majority owner of Joyce International, Inc., a $200 million company engaged in office products distribution and manufacturing. She is a recognized authority on services marketing, and her award-winning articles have been published in the *Harvard Business Review* and the *Journal of Marketing,* as well as in a number of top-selling books. In 1994, Shostack was the first recipient of the Career Contributions Award of the American Marketing Association. She is a summa cum laude graduate of the University of Cincinnati and holds an M.B.A. from Harvard Business School.

Rajendra S. Sisodia, Ph.D., is Associate Professor of Business at George Mason University, in Fairfax, Virginia. Before joining GMU, he was Assistant Professor of Marketing at Boston University. Dr. Sisodia has an M. Phil. and a Ph.D. in Marketing & Business Policy from Columbia University. His research, teaching and consulting expertise spans the areas of marketing strategy and business impacts of information technology. Dr. Sisodia has published over forty articles in conference proceedings and journals such as *Harvard Business Review* and *Journal of Business Strategy.*

Sybil F. Stershic is President of Quality Service Marketing, a marketing consulting firm specializing in service quality management training and marketing planning for service and nonprofit organizations. Stershic has extensive experience in services marketing, having held key management positions in advertising, marketing communications, and sales at several commercial banks ranging from $500 million to more than $2 billion in assets. She also served as an instructor of both marketing and management communications at Lehigh University, and is serving her third term on the international board of directors of the American Marketing Association, where she is currently Vice President of Marketing Management.

Harold J. Steudel, Ph.D., P.E., is president and founder of H.J. Steudel & Associates, Inc., an international consulting company. In addition, he is a professor of industrial engineering at the University of Wisconsin–Madison, where he is active in research and teaching and serves as the convener for the Quality Engineering Program. He has more than 40 published papers and is author of *Manufacturing in the Nineties: How to Become a Mean, Lean, World-Class Competitor.*

Jack Trout is president of Trout & Partners, a marketing strategy firm based in Greenwich, Connecticut. His clients include IBM, Burger King, Chase Manhattan, Xerox, Merck, Proctor & Gamble, and other Fortune 500 companies. Trout was instrumental in developing the vital approach to marketing known as "positioning." Prior to forming his own consulting firm, Trout worked with Al Ries for more than 26 years at Trout & Ries. Together, Trout and Ries have co-authored a number of industry classics and bestsellers, including *Positioning: The Battle for Your Mind; Marketing Warfare;* and *Bottom-Up Marketing.* Their latest book, *The*

22 Immutable Laws of Marketing, outlines the basic reasons marketing programs succeed or fail.

Arthur B. VanGundy, Ph.D., is Professor of Communications at the University of Oklahoma, owner of the consulting firm VanGundy & Associates, Inc., and an associate of New Product Resources, Inc. He has written nine books on creativity and problem solving, and has spoken at numerous conferences and professional meetings in the United States and abroad. VanGundy's consulting clients have included Carrier Corporation, Xerox, Monsanto. Kerr-McGee Chemical, Air-Canada, McNeil Consumer Products (the "Tylenol" people), Eveready Battery, The American Chemical Society, Hallmark Cards, Mitsubishi Heavy Industries America, Hershey Foods, S.C. Johnson & Sons Company (Johnson Wax), Wisconsin Gas, Wyeth-Ayerst Pharmaceutical, the Singapore Civil Service Institute, and the Singapore Institute of Standards and Industrial Research. VanGundy holds a B.A. in psychology, an M.S. in personnel psychology, and a Ph.D. in education.

Rajan Varadarajan is Foley's Professor of Retailing and Marketing at Texas A&M University, and editor of the *Journal of Marketing.* Dr. Varadarajan's interests are corporate, business, and marketing strategy; marketing management; and global competitive strategy. He is author of more than 60 referred journal articles, and is co-author of *Contemporary Perspectives on Strategic Market Planning.* Dr. Varadarajan received his M.A. in industrial management from the Indian Institute of Technology, Madras, India, and his Ph.D. in business administration from the University of Massachusetts, Amherst.

Terry Vavra is Associate Professor of Marketing at the Lubin School of Business at Pace University in New York. Dr. Vavra is a specialist in customer retention strategies, and is author of the book *Aftermarketing: How To Keep Customers for Life through Relationship Marketing.* In addition to his teaching, he also serves as the president of Marketing Metrics, Inc., a consulting and customer retention firm located in Paramus, New Jersey. His clients include Cellular One, Dentsu Inc., Ferrari, IBM, Motorola, Rolls-Royce, and Seiko Instruments. Dr. Vavra is regularly sought as a speaker for international seminars, and has spoken on American marketing techniques to Canadian, French, Japanese, South American, and British audiences.

Judith Waldrop has been research editor of *American Demographics* magazine since 1987. Her writing has been honored by the American Society of Business Press Editors, the American Diabetes Association, the National Religious Public Relations Council, the National Easter Seal Society and American Association of Disability Communicators, and others. She began writing on seasonal variations in consumer markets in 1988 and this was the topic of her first book, *The Seasons of Business.* Prior to coming to *American Demographics,* Ms. Waldrop worked for ten years as a city planner. She holds an MPA from Florida Atlantic University and BGS from Auburn University at Montgomery.

Steven F. Walker is President/CEO of Walker Direct Marketing, L.P., a subsidiary of the Indianapolis based Walker Group of Companies. Walker Group is a 54 year old management information holding company comprised of six separate entities which together account for over $40 million in sales. Walker has spent the last ten years serving the Walker organization in a variety of capacities, including operations management, account management, sales, marketing, analysis, and consulting. He has also published articles and given speeches about marketing research, telemarketing, and database marketing to various industry associations and groups. In 1990, he was instrumental in the founding of Walker Direct as Walker Group's entry into the database marketing industry.

Index

About the Editor

The editor, Jeff Heilbrunn, has been involved in marketing for over 20 years. He has held marketing positions with Cook Electric (Northern Telecom), Quasar Electronics, and the National Safety Council. As President of the American Marketing Association, he came into contact with many of the greatest thinkers in marketing, leading to the conception of this work. Jeff is currently the President of The NOW Group Ltd., of Crystal Lake, Illinois, a marketing consulting and sales representation organization.

American Marketing Association

The American Marketing Association, the world's largest and most comprehensive professional association of marketers, has over 40,000 members worldwide and over 500 chapters throughout North America. It sponsors 25 major conferences per year, covering topics ranging from the latest trends in customer satisfaction measurement to business-to-business and services marketing, to attitude research and sales promotion. The AMA publishes 9 major marketing publications, including *Marketing Management*, a quarterly magazine aimed at marketing managers, and dozens of books addressing special issues, such as relationship marketing, marketing research, and entrepreneurial marketing for small and home-based businesses. Let the AMA be your strategy for success.

For further information on the American Marketing Association, call TOLL FREE at 1-800-AMA-1150.

Or write to
American Marketing Association
250 S. Wacker Drive, Suite 200
Chicago, Illinois 60606
(312) 648-0536
(312) 993-7542 FAX